A Primer for
Health Care Ethics
Essays for a Pluralistic Society

A Primer for
Health Care Ethics
Essays for a Pluralistic Society

Jean deBlois, C.S.J.
Patrick Norris, O.P.
Kevin O'Rourke, O.P.

GEORGETOWN UNIVERSITY PRESS / WASHINGTON, D.C.

Georgetown University Press, Washington, D.C. 20007
© 1994 by Georgetown University Press. All rights reserved.
Printed in the United States of America.
10 9 8 7 6 5 4 3 2 1   1994
THIS VOLUME IS PRINTED ON ACID-FREE OFFSET BOOK PAPER.

Library of Congress Cataloging-in-Publication Data

De Blois, Jean.
   A primer for health care ethics : essays for a pluralistic society
/ Jean deBlois, Patrick Norris, Kevin O'Rourke.
      p. cm.
      1. Medical ethics. 2. Medical ethics—Case studies.   I. Norris,
Patrick, .   II. O'Rourke, Kevin.   III. Title.
R724.D3826   1994
174'.2—dc20
ISBN 0-87840-562-3 (pbk.)   94-11005

Contents

Introduction

Health Care Ethics: A Primer for a Pluralistic Society is a collection of essays originally written for students and professors at the Saint Louis University Health Sciences Center (SLUHSC) as one element of an educational program. The essays are written monthly by the staff of the Center for Health Care Ethics, often in response to questions of health care ethics being discussed in the media. At the suggestion of several of our students and colleagues, we are making the essays available to an even larger audience.

The wisdom of such an enterprise arises from changes in our society. During the past few years, health care ethics has become "everybody's business." The ethical implications of such issues as genetic engineering, assisted suicide, surrogate motherhood, in vitro fertilization, and the AIDS epidemic go beyond the research laboratory, the hospital, and the long term care center. The ethical decisions made in regard to these contemporary research and medical procedures will determine for years to come what kind of people we shall be and what type of society we shall create.

The time is far past when scientists and health care professionals were the only people responsible for ethical decisions regarding research and health care. To paraphrase the famous proverb concerning the responsibility for decisions about war, health care ethics is too important to be left in the hands of scientists and health care professionals. Thus, although we stress the responsibilities of scientists and health care professionals in these essays and articles, we realize that these issues dramatically affect all persons in society. We address these reflections to a wide spectrum of society, realizing that people with many different talents must be involved in the decision-making process that will direct medical research and health care.

Though sponsored by the Society of Jesus (the Jesuits) and thus a Catholic institution, SLUHSC attracts faculty and students from many different ethnic and religious backgrounds. The people of SLUHSC are a pluralistic community similar to our society at large. Hence these essays, while not in conflict with Catholic teaching, are written for a pluralistic community.

Because the essays are designed for a pluralistic audience does not imply that they are without logical foundation, principle, or certitude. Health care ethics founded on personal opinion, emotional reactions, or an erroneous concept of the human person does more harm than good. Rather, these essays are based upon two objective realities: (1) the functions that human persons have in common; and (2) the goals of health care as evidenced in the profession-al-patient relationship. Hence, in the essays one will find frequent references to the physiological, psychological, social, and spiritual functions of the human person. Moreover, it will become clear that while health care in the strict sense is concerned with only the first two functions, it must respect the other two. The mutual responsibility of persons in the professional-patient relationship and the desire to heal physiological and psychological functions while respecting social and spiritual values will also be a theme. Though these essays are directed toward a pluralistic community, we draw upon a very definite concept of the human person and some precise values and goals of the healing relationship which we believe have brought out the best in people in the health care professions over the centuries.

During the past few years, the type of ethical issue facing health care professionals has changed. While the ethical questions in the past were directed toward medical procedures (for example, informed consent, transplantation of organs, and allowing patients to die), today and in the immediate future the more prominent ethical issues in health care will be social issues: why and how to care for the poor; how to preserve quality of care in the face of government controls and fiscal constraints; how to preserve the values of medicine in the face of efforts to commercialize health care; how to choose which health care services will be offered from the many valuable services available. The reader will notice that many of these more contemporary topics are treated in this collection.

While this collection is not presented as a textbook or a model for logical progression in the science of health care ethics, we hope that it will stimulate critical thinking, promote discussion, foster a reasoned understanding of objec-tive principles and, above all, help people actively involved in health care, as well as people outside the profession to ask the right questions when faced with ethical issues.

The essays are gathered in two general sections with no reference to the time at which they were written. Part one contains those essays examining principles and basic concepts of medical ethics for a pluralistic society. For the most part, essays in section two consider cases that have been prominent in the media. While we do not always seek to solve the cases in question because information sufficient for an informed ethical decision is seldom presented in the media, we do seek to present the principles that should be utilized in answering similar questions that might arise in the course of clinical practice.

Finally, we want to express our gratitude to our colleagues at the Center for Health Care Ethics: Mary Elizabeth Hogan, Robert Barnet, M.D. and Mary McGrath, who often discussed these issues with us, also to Donna Grace Troy and Charlotte Ruzicka who supported our work and helped produce this volume.

PART ONE

Principles for a Pluralistic Society

1: What Is Health Care Ethics?

Ethics is the discipline or science by which we determine which human actions are good and which are bad. If we agree that some actions are good and some are bad, it implies that there is a norm or measure for judging human actions. That is, there must be standards to which good actions will conform and to which bad actions do not conform. In this essay, we shall discuss the standards or norms by which free human actions are judged to be good or bad.

Human beings act in order to fulfill their needs. What are our human needs? While we can enumerate many human needs, some very significant such as food and water, and some not so significant but which make life more pleasant, such as ice cream and television, there are four needs that are most basic or fundamental. The four fundamental needs are:

a. physiological needs, satisfied through food and drink
b. psychological needs, satisfied through sense pleasure, rest and relaxation
c. social needs, satisfied through family, friends, and community
d. creative or spiritual needs, satisfied through knowledge, truth, and love

In order to fulfill these four needs, we have powers or functions: biological, emotional, social, and creative. All the needs and their corresponding human functions are important, but creative needs and functions are most important because they direct the attainment of all human needs. Even creative functions will be dependent to some degree upon physiological function. In sum, the functions by which we fulfill human needs are interdependent. The human functions that enable us to fulfill our needs are conceived most aptly as dimensions of a cube rather than floors of a building.

Our needs, or drives as they are sometimes called, motivate us to pursue objects and activities that will satisfy our fundamental needs. We call the objects or activities that fulfill our needs "goods." When seeking goods that will fulfill the fundamental human needs, we know from experience that a person must be careful to fulfill needs in a balanced manner. That is, when fulfilling a need, one must make sure that fulfilling other needs is still possible. For example, eating appetizing food fulfills my physiological and psychological needs, but if I eat too much, I may get sick and be unable to study for the chemistry examination I have tomorrow. By fulfilling my need for food in an unbalanced manner, I have made it impossible to fulfill my creative

3

need, which is fulfilled by passing the chemistry exam. You have heard of the person who studies so intently that she injures her health. This is another example of fulfilling needs in an unbalanced manner. This need to fulfill human needs in a balanced manner is expressed in the distinction between people who live to eat and people who eat to live.

When a human act achieves the goal of fulfilling a human need in a balanced manner, we call such an action a good action. Moreover, the action is described as having value. If a human act does not fulfill a human need, or fulfills a human need in an unbalanced manner, we call such actions bad actions. Thus, if a person steals food from another, he is performing a bad action because, while he may be fulfilling his physiological need, he is not fulfilling his social needs. Or, if a person fulfills his physiological and psychological needs by drinking beer but drinks so much that he impairs his ability to drive a car safely, he is unable to fulfill his social and creative needs, and hence is performing a bad action, whether or not other persons are injured as a result of his drunkenness.

The free judgments by which one chooses to fulfill his or her basic needs are known as ethical decisions, or decisions of conscience. When making decisions of conscience, difficulties arise most often in regard to social needs. Our desire to fulfill our physiological, psychological, and creative needs usually involves our own well-being. But in order to fulfill our social needs, we must be concerned about the well-being of others; that is, we must respect their needs and rights. Experience teaches us how difficult it is to keep the needs and rights of others in mind as we seek to fulfill our own needs. That is why society devotes so much attention to establishing justice through laws, courts, and police force. But we also know that respecting the rights and needs of others is vitally important because it is the basis for friendship and community, peace and progress.

As we affirm that the purpose of human acts is to fulfill human needs in a balanced manner, we also affirm that when a person fails to act in a balanced manner, he is still trying to do something that he considers to be good. To put it another way, if a person chooses to do something that does not fulfill his needs in a balanced manner, he chooses an action that is subjectively good, but that is objectively evil. The distinction between subjective and objective morality is most important in ethics. This distinction helps us understand the nature of good and evil. A human action that is both objectively and subjectively good is a human act that fulfills a person's needs in a balanced manner. However, an action may be objectively evil, but only subjectively good. This happens when the act is only a partial or apparent good. The error in judgment that leads a person to choose an apparent good rather than a true or balanced good may be due to an intellectual error or to moral weakness. Hence, a person may choose to take the property of another, erroneously thinking it is his own property. If one is not responsible for the ignorance that disposes one to act in this way, it might be considered an evil action objectively speaking, but it is clear that the person taking the property of the other is not doing something evil insofar as the subjective order of morality is concerned. Moral weakness might cause one to choose a partial or apparent good when the opportunity to steal money without being caught causes one to neglect fulfillment of his social needs. If a person decides to steal a large sum of money, he concentrates upon the good that will come to him when he has more money and thinks little about the harm that will come to the people from whom he steals the money. If the thief thinks of his victims at all, he might excuse his violation of human rights by saying, "Anyhow, they won't miss it!" Conflicts regarding moral judgments arise when people, either because of ignorance or moral weakness, do not consider all their human needs when making ethical decisions. When making ethical decisions in regard to health care, for example, the medical team is interested in prolonging life, a physiological good. Patients, however, may have spiritual norms they wish to fulfill. Thus, a patient who is a Jehovah's Witness will seek to fulfill her religious belief that prohibits blood transfusions, even though she may die as a result of her choice. Insofar as she is concerned, she is making a good ethical decision because fulfilling her spiritual need is more important than fulfilling her physiological need. In the mind of the medical team, however, she is making a bad decision because she is thwarting her ability to live and prolong life. Medical teams sometimes try to persuade Jehovah's Witness patients to allow blood transfusions or what is more problematical, will transfuse them if they are comatose. Ethical patient care requires that the medical team realize that fulfilling spiritual needs is more important than fulfilling physiological needs because spiritual needs have the most important place in the levels of human needs.

In order to facilitate ethical decision making, ethical norms have been constructed that express which actions are good and which are bad. These ethical norms are an effort to codify or express the experience that people have had when making individual ethical decisions. Therefore, we have positive ethical norms, such as: "tell the truth," "honor your father and mother," and negative ethical norms, such as: "do not steal" and "do not commit adultery." In most cases, these norms can simply be followed without a great deal of discussion because usually their validity can be easily discerned. But sometimes, more investigation is needed to see if the norm has validity for a particular action; that is, whether or not the particular act in question corresponds to the norm. Thus, the good protected by observing the ethical norm "do not steal" is the good of private property. But could it happen that a person would starve to death if she did not steal some money or food? Is the good of human life more important than the good of private property? Thus, some ethical norms are subject to evaluation when it seems the norm would impose irrational behavior. Another way of stating this is to say: The circumstances in which acts are performed may change the ethical evaluation of the act. Is this true of all ethical norms? Are all ethical norms relative in the sense that circumstances may change the authority of the norm? This issue is highly debated in ethics. As the essays in this volume illustrate, there are some ethical norms that are so important, such as respecting the worth of innocent human life, that they oblige under all conditions and circumstances. But at times the circumstances of an act will have a greater impact upon the morality of the act. For example, determining whether the removal of life support is ethical or unethical depends upon the circumstances that relate to the patient's medical condition. Given the medical condition of the patient, will continued use of a respirator be beneficial for the patient? As we shall see in some of the essays contained in this book, the meaning of the word "benefit" is open to different interpretations.

In the course of history, several general norms have been formulated to guide the ethical practice of medicine. These norms are derived from the experience of physicians and nurses seeking to fulfill the needs of patients and care givers in a balanced manner. Because ethical medicine seeks to fulfill all the needs of the patient, an ethical physician or nurse seeks to do more than keep the patient alive. Some of the norms for the ethical practice of medicine are:

1. Do no harm to the patient.
2. Obtain informed consent from the patient or the proxy.
3. Respect human life and bodily integrity.
4. Tell the truth.
5. Maintain confidentiality, especially concerning harmful facts and information.
6. Respect the faith of the patient.
7. Do not use patients in research projects without their consent.
8. Allow patients to die if life-prolonging therapy is ineffective or imposes an excessive burden.
9. Offer health care because people are in need, not because they can pay for it.

Clearly, when applying these norms, there is often a need to resolve conflicts that arise between different norms; for example, do community needs ever modify the norm to observe confidentiality? It seems so, because cases of venereal disease must be reported to public authorities so that the community may take steps to limit the disease. Or more concretely, how far can we go in observing norm 9 without impeding the effort to provide health care for those who are able to pay for their care? Most of the time, however, these principles can be applied correctly with little discussion about their meaning or applicability.

Taking time to study carefully whether a particular action will fulfill the human needs of a particular person in a balanced manner is a time-consuming and difficult process. For this reason, when making ethical decisions in health care, the medical facts must be obtained, that is, the diagnosis and prognosis must be ascertained. Often the diagnosis and prognosis will not be certain, thus uncertainty is often a factor that makes ethical decisions in health care confusing or difficult. When removing life support, for example, the ethical decision is often made more difficult because the effect of removing the life support is often unknown; will continuing the life support be a benefit for the patient or will continuing it be ineffective or an excessive burden? If some degree of moral certitude cannot be obtained, sound ethical decision making requires that the more cautious action, the action most likely to protect patient benefit, should be followed. After discerning the medical facts, the options for action must be analyzed insofar as patient benefit is concerned. These options must be compared with one another. Unfortunately, perfect options are seldom available. Given the circumstances, the best or better option must be selected. Often the choice of the better or best option will result from a comparison of human needs that will be fulfilled by the particular options. Patient benefit must take into consideration the four basic levels mentioned above. Finally, one option must be selected. Theoretically, the option chosen will not always be the perfect option, objectively speaking, but it should be an option substantiated by moral certitude as the best option under the present circumstances. If a list of options for treating some illnesses are suggested, one may be too expensive or impose excessive burdens. For example, the best treatment for emphysema maybe to move to a warm and dry climate. But not many people have the money to relocate or the inclination to leave friends and family. Thus, an option for treating the emphysema must be chosen that in theory is less effective but is the best hope for cure or palliative care under the circumstances. Given what is known at this time, and given what we can predict about the future, acting in this way seems the best manner to promote the well-being of the patient. This process of decision making is called reasoned analysis or personalism, because it endeavors to bring human reason to the center of ethical decision making and seeks to benefit persons in their quest for human fulfillment.[1]

Sometimes the process of reasoned analysis may be shortened through the use of moral norms, but as explained above, the moral norms themselves will be the subject of reasoned analysis in some particular situations. Because the process of evaluating human needs and determining whether an action fulfills human needs in a balanced manner through reasoned analysis is time-consuming and difficult, there is a tendency among human beings to make ethical decisions through other methods. We offer a brief description of some of these methods and point out the shortcomings of these methods in essay 14. In one way or another, these methods dispose for ethical error because they do not utilize a thorough analysis of the four human needs as an integral part of the process of decision making.

CONCLUSIONS

In conclusion, let us consider a description of the collaborative process of reasoned analysis for making ethical decisions in regard to matters of health care.

1. Discern important medical facts affecting basic needs of the patient.
2. Discern conflicts in fulfilling needs; if no conflicts, probably no ethical problem.
3. Consider the various options for fulfilling patient's needs. If a conflict arises in regard to patient need, consult the patient or proxy.
4. Following the moral principle of informed consent, determine with the patient or proxy which option, here and now, will best fulfill the patient's need in an integrated manner. Ethical principles will usually help in this step of process.
5. If you are morally certain that the option selected is a good ethical decision, follow through with it. If you have serious doubts, confirm your choice by comparing it to other cases and by discussing it with others.

NOTE

1. Benedict Ashley and Kevin O'Rourke, *Health Care Ethics*, 3d ed. (St. Louis: Catholic Health Association, 1989), Chapter 7.

2: Medical Ethics: Search for Principles

Many individuals and professional organizations maintain that ethics committees must be formed in hospitals in order to help answer the questions arising from advanced technology and increased recognition of patient's rights. Even if the committees are confined to a role of educational activities and not given the power to make ethical decisions for others, a practical question arises: What principles will the committee use when deliberating about ethical issues or when trying to formulate policy to be presented to the administration for approval? Drawing together ten people with ten different ethical perspectives might bring chaos rather than consensus. Is there a common understanding of medical ethics that will enable people on ethics committees to function cooperatively and intelligently despite different professions, backgrounds, and religious persuasions?

PRINCIPLES

Medical ethics arises from the relationship between a patient and a physician. The patient goes to a physician seeking health. Health, in this limited sense, is the well-being of physiological and psychological functions. Health is of great value for the patient, but it is not the only value. The patient has values associated with social or spiritual functions as well.

The physician enters the relationship promising to help the patient achieve health. This promise is based upon two assumptions:

1. The physician will strive for competency in the field of medicine.
2. The physician promises to respect the patient as a person. Hence, in addition to the value of health in a limited sense, the other values (social and spiritual) the patient might have will be respected. Thus, the physician agrees to respect the patient's quest for health in the wider sense of the term. This latter respect for social and spiritual aspects arises from the fact that the physician respects the patient as an equal. Although the patient is subordinate or unequal to the physician in medical skill and knowledge, he or she deserves respect as a person of equal worth insofar as the other values of life are concerned.

Often there will be no conflict between the patient's health values and social and spiritual values. In most circumstances patients look upon healing

9

(a physiological or psychological value) as a necessary means for achieving other values in life (social and spiritual). Thus, in most cases, difficult ethical decisions will not be in question because no choice between conflicting values is necessary. Rather, these routine cases call only for protection of the patient's basic rights as a human being (e.g., the right to be informed, the right to maintain one's reputation).

But in some cases there will be a conflict between maintaining or restoring health (achieving psychological or physiological values) and achieving social or spiritual values. For example, an aging patient suffering from a terminal illness may decide that he or she would be better off spiritually if life-prolonging therapy were withdrawn and death allowed to ensue. A person might believe that divine law prohibits the use of blood transfusions even if they would prolong life. In cases of this nature, the conflict must be settled by treatment that respects the patient's values. The ethical basis for the patient's right to choose the type of treatment is the fact that as a human being the patient is equal to the physician. When entering the healing relationship the patient does not surrender personal responsibility for determining which values are more important in a given situation.

In like manner, the physician does not surrender his or her value system when entering the healing relationship. Thus, there may be difficult ethical decisions for physicians to make as well; for example, is it contrary to my value system to allow a patient to die when I know life could be prolonged? Should I operate on the person who refuses blood transfusion knowing there is increased danger of death? Hence, the medical relationship seeks to achieve health but does not posit health as the ultimate human value for patient or physician.

DISCUSSION

The goal of healing the patient in accord with his or her value system serves as the touchstone of ethical medical practice in particular and of health care in general. Of course, other factors should be considered in medical and health care; for example, economic and societal factors enter into the offering of medical and health care. These economic and social factors are especially prominent today with the national focus on cost-effectiveness, competition, and reducing the use of health care facilities. Although these economic and social factors must be considered by the ethical physician or hospital adminis-trator, they must never be allowed to dominate the practice of medical care or health care. If they do, then a perversion of values occurs, and physicians and other health care professionals betray the trust of patients and their own integrity. Resisting the pressure to make economic or societal factors the basis for decision making will be difficult for ethics committees as well as for physicians and other health care professionals.

From the nature of the healing relationship and the presuppositions mentioned above, the general principle of medical ethics can be deduced. For example, in order to enable patients to express their value systems and to ensure they are treated as equals, informed consent is required; informed consent gives rise to the principle that health care professionals should tell the truth; because the patient's reputation is of great value, the principle of confidentiality is posited.

Although these and other principles of medical ethics are deduced from the nature of the physician-patient relationship, they should not be applied as though they were straitjackets determining every particular decision. In practice, two patients may be treated differently because each might have a different value system. Thus, medical ethics is not relativistic or circumstantial because it does have valid general principles. But it is flexible because these general principles must be applied to individual patients who have different needs and value systems. Facing a choice between death and severely debilitated survival, one person might choose life-prolonging therapy; another might choose only pain-relieving therapy.

CONCLUSION

Ethics committees can be helpful if the people serving on them have a common understanding of the nature of medical ethics. Judging from the literature on the subject, however, ethics committees often seem to be promoted as a means of defusing the moral responsibility of avoiding malpractice litigation or of removing the anguish from difficult ethical decisions. There is no way to make difficult ethical decisions easy. People serving on ethics committees would do well to ponder constantly the question: Do we have a common understanding of medical ethics?

3: The Values Inherent in Medical Care

Values influence—and in many cases determine—human behavior; they give direction and meaning not only to individual actions but also to our personalities. What values are associated with health care? Are any values so closely associated with medical care that to neglect them would frustrate the effort to offer that care? In order to study these questions adequately, we shall consider the concepts of health, human function, and health care.

PRINCIPLES

Health and health care are interdependent; hence, to understand the values associated with health care, one must possess a clear notion of human health. Ask the physician, nurse, or hospital administrator, "What is health?" and you are liable to receive a blank look in reply. Henrik Blum concludes a searching analysis of the concept of health with the brief formula, "Health is the state of being in which an individual does the best with the capacities he has, and acts in ways that maximize his system."[1] Because a human being is an organism, it is an open system. Hence, in maintaining balance or homeostasis, a person is continually relating to the environment. For our purposes, then, we conceive of health as optimal human functioning, which implies not only an internal harmony and consistency of function, but also the capacity of the organism to maintain itself in its environment.

What is conveyed by the term *human function?* Human beings are born with the need to eat; because we feel hunger (the need for nutrition in order to survive), we perform the function of eating. We have a capacity for knowledge; because we feel a need for truth in order to understand and fulfill our purpose in life, we perform the function of learning. It is widely acknowledged that there are four categories of human needs and corresponding functions: (1) biological or physiological; (2) psychological; (3) social; and (4) spiritual or creative.

Given these basic needs and functions, it is extremely important to discern how they are related, since this relationship will provide a blueprint for the quest for health and the limits of medical care. Is one function more important than another? If so, it will contribute more to health. Are the relationships among the various functions cooperative or competitive? Can one function be sacrificed for another without impairing the individual's health?

12

These four functions are not stories in a building, one on top of the other, but rather interrelated dimensions of human activity. Just as the length, height, and depth of a cube can be distinguished conceptually for sake of study, but not separated in reality, so the four functions of the human act are interconnected. Every truly human act involves all four functions. A human spiritual act, whether it be the creative act of a scientist or the loving act of a parent, involves a biological, psychological, and social function at the same time. True, one type of function will predominate in a human act, but all types will be present.

The task of the creative function is to integrate the biological, psychological, and social functions. Thus creative functions are the deepest, most central, and most complex. At the same time, however, these activities are rooted in and dependent upon the other functions in a network of interrelations. One cannot think unless one's brain is physiologically sound. Even though interdependent, each function is to a certain extent independent—structurally and functionally differentiated—so that when help in restoring function is needed, each function is served by a different discipline. To restore the physiological function of bone structure, for instance, an orthopedist is called; for psychological function, a psychologist or psychiatrist is needed; for the social function, a social counselor or lawyer is required; for the creative-spiritual function, a teacher or spiritual director is called for.

The ultimate goal of health care then is an optimally functioning human person. Notice that this concept is richer and more complex than the ultimate goal put forward for health care by many ethicists: the autonomy of the person.[2]

DISCUSSION

Clearly, physicians and all other medical care professionals must be concerned proximately and primarily with healing the physiological and psychological functions. However, their efforts at restoring these functions must be performed with the awareness of the interrelatedness of all human functions. Thus, the ultimate goal of health care must be health in the fuller sense: the coordinated functioning of all human powers. Physicians who do not realize the interrelatedness of all human functions might think they have the right to make all decisions for the patient; health planning might be directed only to the betterment of physiological functions without regard for their relation to psychological, social, or spiritual functions.

Even though patients present themselves in a wounded state of health, as a result of which they have lost some degree of self-determination, the patient's power to make his or her own decisions must be respected by the physician and all other persons in health care. Because of the good in question, and because there is a need to respect the patient's spiritual integrity, a specific type of relationship arises between the physician and the patient, known familiarly as the professional relationship. The heart of this relationship is an avowal (*professio*) that one person is willing to help another person attain an important human good while at the same time respecting that person's personal worth and dignity. Given the service value in the relationship between the professional and the person in need of help, it is evident that the relationship must be built on trust. This is especially true in medicine, where the patient's vulnerability is multidimensional and the patient-physician relationship is intrinsically imbalanced.

If our brief account of the values inherent in the medical relationship is accurate, then it is clear why profit cannot be the primary basis of any profession but must be considered a secondary and highly variable feature. Traditionally, a principle fundamental to all professions has been that the professional must be ready to give services free to those who are in need but cannot pay. Indeed, official codes of medical ethics usually state that fees should be adjusted to the ability of the patient to pay.

In view of the foregoing, the following value statements are normative for individuals and corporations involved in health care:

1. Those offering medical care must remember and respect the worth and higher functions of the individual; this implies something more than mere "autonomy."
2. The overriding purpose of medical care must be a desire to serve those whose physiological or psychological health is impaired in order to enable them to lead a better life.
3. The patient-physician relationship must be permeated by trust.
4. Medical care should not be considered a commodity, something to be bought or sold in a market system, because it is a precious and vital good to which no price can be attached and because it is prerequisite to the attainment of other human goods as well as to the pursuit of a meaningful life.

NOTES

1. Henrik Blum, *Expanding Health Care Horizons: From General Systems Concept of Health Care to a National Policy*, Oakland, Third Party Publications, 1983, p. 27.

2. Charles J. Dougherty, *Ideal Fact and Medicine,* (New York: University Press of America, 1985), 66 ff.

4: Can We Agree?

Medical history shows that in every age, medical practice has been embroiled not only in scientific controversies, but also in ethical ones. The introduction of vaccination, the use of quinine, the administration of anesthesia, performing heart transplants, and defining death through lack of brain activity—all produced serious ethical controversies. Many of these ethical issues continue to this day and are hotly debated. The unfortunate side effect of ethical debate is that people often become discouraged with reaching an agreement. Thus, they separate into diverse groups and ultimately converse only with people with whom they agree. Health care professionals often wonder why such sharp differences exist in the realm of medical ethics.

PRINCIPLES

Ethical questions are inevitably controversial for various reasons, including the following:

1. Ethical questions are complex, involving many different factors; it is thus possible to get different results by emphasizing different aspects of a problem. In the abortion issue, for instance, one group emphasizes the rights of the mother, and the other group emphasizes the rights of the unborn child, and little dialogue results.
2. Ethics deals with profound and mysterious issues of human life such that our knowledge of values involved is incomplete and always open to further study.
3. Ethical matters cannot be completely universalized into rules because they involve the individual and individual situations, so there is always a difficulty in applying general rules to concrete cases. Thus, ethics is not relativistic because all human beings have much in common. But applying principles to individual cases is more than a mathematical procedure.
4. Ethics treats questions not only of fact but also of value. Values influence both our thought and our feeling and will. They involve an essential element of subjectivity as well as an objective foundation in human experience.
5. Ethical decisions not only affect abstract questions, but also change our personal lives directly. Because such change is painful, it is difficult not to be prejudiced in ethical judgment, since "no person is a good judge

15

in his or her own case." Usually people try to defend their prior ethical
positions rather than subject them to criticism.

6. Ethical perceptions depend on our concrete experience, and all persons
or groups have their own history and special culture, which profoundly
influence their ethical outlook. Thus, we are intimately involved in
our ethical viewpoints.

7. Fundamental to all particular ethical judgments is the religion or its
equivalent philosophy of life with its value systems to which the
individual or group consciously or unconsciously adheres.

8. Besides the difficulties that arise from our human finitude are the
difficulties that have their origin in what is called human sinfulness,
which darkens our understanding and distorts our motivation. Whether
this sinfulness is the result of human history embodied in social structures or of our own individual contribution to this human condition
is, in a sense, immaterial. It is present in our lives, whether we look
on it as primarily social or primarily personal.

DISCUSSION

In view of these difficulties, how are we to develop a satisfactory and mature
approach to ethical controversies in medical discussion? A hint of an answer
can be derived from the psychological studies of Jean Piaget and Lawrence
Kohlberg, which have shown that in most groups of adults there are persons
at different levels of development in ethical thinking, corresponding to the
phases through which a child must pass to full moral maturity. These phases
can be summarized in three main levels:

1. The small child tends to make decisions on the basis of the immediate
consequences of an action (i.e., rewards and punishments).

2. The growing child begins to make decisions more and more on the
basis of social approval of parents or peers. Conformity to group norms
becomes paramount, and satisfactions can be delayed and suffering
incurred to achieve approval of others.

3. Moral maturity is marked by an increasing internalization and independence of such moral judgment. Decisions are now made on the basis
of personal standards, and the standards of society become subject to
criticism. The adult acts primarily for self-approval, even at the cost
of disapproval by the group.

Most ethical controversies seem to be carried on largely at the second
level. The debaters each proceed on the assumption that the value system of
their group, whether it be that of a social class, a professional elite, or a
church, is self-evident, and they make little or no effort to understand the

viewpoint of opponents who live within other competing value systems. This mindset has been demonstrated by various groups within the field of health care as they disagree over ethical issues; however, it is also demonstrated by health care professionals as a group as they disagree with other groups in society over values. For example, associations representing health care professionals seem continually at odds with associations representing people interested in reducing health care costs.

In the United States, the four main value systems involved in most public debates are: humanism, Judaism, Catholicism, and Protestantism with their many subsystems. Because each of these groups rests its arguments on assumptions the others do not share, public controversies on medical-moral matters such as abortion or therapy for the dying tend to end in stalemate. However, with patience and fairness it may sometimes be possible to pursue a question to the third and mature level of ethical thinking, in which it becomes possible to subject even these assumptions to examination, reinterpretation, and, we hope, eventual ecumenical convergence. Ethical discourse of this nature requires patience, understanding, and generosity.

5: Informed Consent

Informed consent is never out of the news. Despite the emphasis given to this component of ethical medical care, difficulties in obtaining informed consent have been expressed over the years. For example, a few years ago, one author stated:

> Within one day of signing consent forms for chemotherapy, radiation therapy, or surgery, 200 cancer patients completed a test of their recall of the material in the consent explanation and filled out a questionnaire regarding their opinions of its purpose, content, and implications. Only 60 percent understood the purpose and nature of the procedure, and only 55 percent correctly listed even one major risk or complication . . . only 40 percent had read the form carefully . . . and only 27 percent could name one alternative treatment.[1]

Often the problem *is* the consent forms. A study of consent forms from five representative hospitals revealed that the readability of all five were approximately equivalent to that of material intended for upper division under-graduates or graduate students. Four of the five norms were written at the level of a scientific journal, and the fifth at the level of a specialized academic magazine.

Our purpose is not to confirm or to deny the conclusions in the above-mentioned studies; they speak for themselves. They also offer, however, an opportunity to review some thoughts about informed consent and to discuss why it is necessary for ethical decision making.

PRINCIPLES

The ethical and legal requirements for informed consent are (1) information, (2) comprehension, and (3) voluntariness.

1. The specific *information* that should be provided for the patient concerns the purpose of the procedure, anticipated risks and benefits, alternative procedures, and hoped-for results. Information should never be withheld for the purpose of eliciting consent, and truthful answers should always be given to direct questions. If a research project is in question, then information may be withheld provided the subject is informed that some information will not be revealed until

18

the research is completed and that no direct harm results from withholding the information.

2. *Comprehension* of the conveyed knowledge is a requirement more complex than it might seem at first. Because subjects' capability to understand varies so greatly, the material must be adapted to the subjects' capacities. Health care professionals are responsible for ascertaining that the subject has comprehended the information, especially if the risk is serious. If the patient cannot comprehend, then some third party, usually a family member but sometimes a person appointed by the court, should be asked to act in the patient's best interest. Some have maintained that comprehension of difficult medical terms is not possible for the ordinary person, but research has shown that persons unfamiliar with medical terms can understand and retain explanations about medical procedures if the explanations are well-planned and given in plain language.

3. *Voluntariness* implies that the person understands the situation clearly and that no coercion or undue influence is exercised by the health care professional. However, it is often difficult to determine where justifiable persuasion ends and undue influence begins. The health care professional who believes that some particular treatment is better for the patient should state his or her conviction but should also explain clearly the reason for this opinion. Voluntariness does not imply that the patient will be free from all pressure or persuasion in a given circumstance. For example, a person with an inflamed appendix is limited insofar as freedom of choice is concerned. But voluntariness does imply that, over and above the limitations arising from the circumstances, no external coercion or moral manipulation is present.

DISCUSSION

Some think that informed consent is required only for research protocols or for experimental procedures. Actually, informed consent is required for any action that would affect a person's physiological, psychological, or moral integrity. Why is informed consent so important? Does it merely help avoid malpractice, or does it fulfill an important human need?

Respect for persons, one of the most basic ethical principles, is carried out in practice through informed consent. The patient's right to informed consent arises from the conviction that human beings are responsible for their own actions and their own destinies. They must be treated as equals and allowed to make the important decisions of life for themselves whenever possible. Only in this way will they be able to reach their full potential as human beings. Although the health care professional offers help to the patient, the health care professional is not given the right to make decisions for the patient nor to manipulate the patient. Health care professionals will dispose for the total and integrative betterment of the human beings whom they serve only if they are careful in observing the requirements of informed consent.

NOTE

1. B. Cassileth, "Informed Consent—Why Are Its Goals Imperfectly Realized," *New England Journal of Medicine* 302 (1980): 896; and T. Grunder, "On Readability of Surgical Consent Forms," *New England Journal of Medicine* 302 (1980): 900.

6: Proxy Consent: Deciding for Others

Four well-publicized and highly controverted legal decisions determining medical treatment for people no longer able to decide for themselves (Quinlan, Saikewicz, Spring, and Fox) call attention to the meaning of proxy consent. These cases provide a framework for reviewing the ethical norms for this type of consent and for commenting briefly on the aforementioned decisions.

Whenever possible, informed consent on the part of the subject is ethically and legally necessary for every medical treatment and research project. Sometimes, however, the subject is not able to give informed consent. For example, an aged person in a coma, an infant, or a fetus cannot perform the rational act necessary for informed consent even though he or she may require some medical treatment. In such cases, another person is called on to offer informed consent: this is called proxy or vicarious consent.

PRINCIPLES

Although proxy consent is often identified with personal informed consent, the two are quite different. Informed consent by a proxy is not a subspecies of personal informed consent; rather, it is a substitute for personal informed consent and is sought when acquiring personal informed consent is impossible. For the ethical and legal use of proxy informed consent, two conditions must be present: (1) the patient or research subject cannot offer informed consent; and (2) the person offering the proxy consent must determine what the incompetent person would have decided were he or she able to make the ethical decision. This second condition is difficult to ascertain and may be subject to dispute.

Decisions of proxy consent should be made in view of the good of the individual patient, not for the higher good of society, nor for a class good, because this would amount to manipulation of the person. When deciding on the treatment for a comatose person dying of cancer, for example, the proxy must seek to determine what the patient would decide if able to make the decision. What would benefit people other than the patient should not be considered unless it can be assumed reasonably that this would have been the consideration of the patient. Hence, parents of a neonate with serious birth anomalies may not say, "Let the baby die; he will be a burden to us." Rather, they must make a decision in accord with the good of the child, weighing

21

especially the fact that, in most cases, we judge life to be a gift worth preserving, even if living may involve working with handicaps or infirmities. Because some parents abuse their rights to decide for their children, there is a trend to question the rights of parents to make proxy judgments and to insist on a better system of checks and balances than exists presently.

DISCUSSION

Because of the nature of a proxy judgment, the person given the right to make such a judgment for another should be one who knows the person well and who has a loving concern for his or her well-being. Usually, then, the person who is presumed to have a legal and ethical right to make a proxy judgment is the parent, spouse, or next of kin; however, others such as physicians and ethical or spiritual counselors, should be consulted.

The presumption that a parent, spouse, or relative will judge rightly is especially strong because of the bond of love that unites such a person to the patient. But of course, this is not an absolute presumption. It may yield to a contrary fact. Thus, if the person who has the right to make this decision decides on something that does not seem to be in accord with the good of the patient, other responsible people may challenge the decision of the proxy and bring the matter before an ethics committee and, in some cases, before the civil authority. Physicians, nurses, and hospital administrators who determine with good reason that the proxy is not acting in accord with the patient's best interests have the ethical, and sometimes legal obligation to intervene. If the case cannot be settled within the family and hospital community, the authority of the courts is often invoked. The legal decisions mentioned in the introduction are examples of the court's intervening in the treatment of a patient. Unfortunately, in the Saikewicz, Spring, and Fox decisions, the courts determined that only the legal authority can act as proxy for removing life-sustaining equipment in life or death situations. These decisions arrogate to public authority matters that belong in the private and personal domain and show a general lack of trust for loved ones to interpret the wishes of a comatose and, in these cases, dying person.

CONCLUSION

The aforementioned legal decisions were reached because the courts based their thinking on the notion that preserving life is an absolute good, and thus the courts "have no choice but to intervene and examine each case on an individual patient by patient basis."[1] Although preserving life is a highly valued good, and although when doubt exists, the proxy should decide in favor of prolonging life, in some circumstances the proxy may determine ethically to allow a person to die because the therapy is ineffective or imposes a serious burden. For example, when prolonging life would not serve any human purpose or would impose an intolerable burden on the patient, the decision to withhold or remove life-supporting therapy may be made as long as the normal care due a sick person is maintained. Thus, it seems that a more nuanced ethical evaluation would have kept all of these cases out of court in the first place. Be that as it may, the usurpation by the courts of ethical decision making can be viewed only with great alarm.

NOTE

1. *Eichner v Dillon*, 426 NY State 2d., 517, 550 (App. Div. 1980).

7: Informed Consent and the Purpose of Medicine

The principle of informed consent is accepted widely as the norm that should guide decision making in the context of the patient-physician relationship. In brief, the principle requires the following: The physician must give sufficient *information* about proposed medical interventions to the person deciding about the use of the proposed interventions. The physician must help the person *understand* the information so that the decision made will be consistent with the person's own beliefs, goals, and values. The physician must ensure that the decision to consent to or refuse the proposed intervention is a *free and voluntary* choice by the person. From an ethical perspective, observance of the principle helps to foster the appropriate goals of the care-giving relationship in two ways. First, the principle focuses attention on the respect that is due to persons with regard to their right to choose their own goals and to make decisions to achieve those goals. Second, by defining the roles and responsibilities of the persons in the care-giving relationship the importance of a collaborative approach in making decisions about health care is emphasized. Insofar as it functions in this manner, observing the principle of informed consent is crucial to striving for the appropriate goals of medicine. But misunderstanding of the principle threatens to undermine the legitimate purposes of medicine and to compromise the ethical integrity of individual practitioners as well.

INFORMED CONSENT AND THE GOOD OF THE PERSON

Ethical or right action is action that seeks to respond to human needs in a way that promotes the "good" or fulfillment of the person. Within the specific context of health care, doing what is "good" for the person means doing that which contributes to the integrated functioning of the person so that the person is able to pursue life's goods and goals. This concept is also referred to as fulfilling the mission of life. When making decisions about the use or non-use of medical therapies the primary question to be answered is: Will use of this therapy enable me to pursue the goods and goals of life, i.e., my mission in life, to some degree? Consider, for example, the use of hemodialysis for a person suffering from renal failure. The fact that the procedure can keep the person alive may not sufficiently justify its use insofar as the person is concerned. Rather, the ability of the person to participate in life in a way that is fulfilling for the person is the norm for measuring the acceptability of

24

chronic hemodialysis. Within this context, the ethical principle of informed consent identifies the conditions necessary for making decisions that contribute to the person's good, which help the person pursue the mission of life.

MISUNDERSTANDING OF THE PRINCIPLE OF INFORMED CONSENT

In what appears to be an extension of the pervasive societal fascination with individual freedom and liberty, many seek to define informed consent exclusively in terms of personal autonomy. As a result, regard for the principle of informed consent is thought by many physicians to require nothing more than a simple solicitation of and compliance with what the individual patient (or surrogate) *wants or desires*. This interpretation reflects the widely held societal belief that the "self" is all important and is defined solely by "its ability to choose its own values."[1] Because personal preferences, which are highly idiosyncratic, are held to delimit the self many conclude that "each self constitutes its own moral universe."[2] Thus, self-fulfillment, according to this opinion, is a highly individualistic endeavor. Two conclusions follow from this opinion. First, there is no objective basis for determining what *is good or fulfilling* with regard to persons. Hence, there are no objective criteria that can serve to guide or provide limits to individual decision making and choice. Second, the person exists in isolation. Relationship with others is desirable only insofar as the relationship furthers personal wants or desires. Thus, there is no basis for concern about the needs or good of the community of persons when seeking to achieve one's own good. When the meaning and requirements of informed consent are interpreted in this individualistic way, the reality of consent as "a shared process of decision making"[3] is nullified. What results are situations in which the physician becomes the mere instrument of the autonomous patient (or of the patient's surrogate). Medical decisions, selected from an individualistic perspective, may indeed be harmful to the patient insofar as he is a being with social responsibilities.

Consider the often cited case of the irreversibly comatose person maintained on life support because "this is what the person wanted." Or consider the case of Janet Adkins who, upon learning that she was in the early stages of Alzheimer's disease, requested the help of a physician in bringing about her own death. In complying with Mrs. Adkins request, the physician argued that his action was justified because the physician's role is limited to carrying out the autonomously expressed wants and desires of the patient. In neither example is there any recognition that the physician has a responsibility to contribute to an understanding of *what is good* from the more objective social perspective and to help in determining *appropriate means* to promote the good. In other words, in both examples, the physician's role is limited to that of a technician.

INFORMED CONSENT RIGHTLY UNDERSTOOD

In seeking to understand what the principle of informed consent requires of the physician, consideration of the patient's personal autonomy is important. However, the patient's autonomy is neither the primary nor the sole consideration. Something more is needed. Correct understanding of informed consent requires and depends on an appreciation of the following: First, the "good" that is sought for an individual person is not only a personal good; we receive our concept of the good from society as well. What is good for the person is that which responds to human needs. But these needs are given with the nature of the human and are shared by all persons. Hence, it is within the community of persons that we come to understand what *is good*, what contributes to human fulfillment. Accordingly, our society seeks to prevent suicide because we know that suicide is not an appropriate response to human need. It is not an act that promotes the social good of the person. Suicide is harmful both to the individual person and to the community of persons as well. Second, when assessing the ability of a proposed medical therapy to enable an individual person to pursue the mission of life, the assessment must take place in a societal context. This is required because the person pursues life's mission as a member of community. Thus, the understanding of informed consent as a shared process of decision making is quite appropriate. It is in light of this understanding that the role of the physician is correctly interpreted.

CONCLUSION

In the care-giving relationship and in the decision-making process the physician does provide technical expertise and must be competent in doing so. But the physician enters the relationship not just as technician but as a fellow member of the community of persons. Thus, the physician is responsible to help the patient discern what *is good* in light of the community's understanding of the good. In addition, the physician must help the person assess actions taken to promote that good not only insofar as those actions affect the individual person but also as they affect the community.

NOTES

1. Robert Bellah, et al. *Habits of the Heart* (New York: Harper & Row, 1985), 75.
2. Ibid., 78.
3. President's Commission, *Making Health Care Decisions* (Washington, DC: U.S. Government Printing Office, 1982), 15ff.

8: Telling the Truth to Patients

"What to tell the patient" has been considered one of the more difficult and delicate ethical questions for health care professionals. In the not too distant past, some physicians and other health care professionals thought that the less patients knew about their condition, the better would be their chances of recovery. Some health care professionals would even withhold information of impending death, fearing that such knowledge might lead a person to despair. Because of an awakened moral sense on the part of health care professionals and a sharper realization that patients have legal and moral rights that must be respected, there is now a much greater tendency to be open and honest concerning patients' conditions, the purpose of the proposed treatment, and the treatment prognosis. *The Patient's Bill of Rights* of the American Hospital Association states:

> The patient has the right to obtain from the physician complete current information concerning diagnosis, treatment, and prognosis in terms the patient can be reasonably expected to understand.

PRINCIPLES

Clearly, information on serious sickness or impending death must be furnished even if the individual does not ask for it. Legal precedent as well as moral concern prompts this realization. Hence, physicians and other health care professionals may not defend their lack of communication by pleading that the patient did not wish to know and did not ask questions. In some hospitals, a patients' representative helps patients understand their situation, especially when surgery is anticipated. Whenever possible, the leader of the health care team, the physician, should be involved in explaining the situation to the patient.

Although health care professionals usually respect patients' rights insofar as providing the proper information, difficult situations often arise and health care professionals hesitate to tell patients their true condition. For example, patients with serious cases of cancer might become despondent and even suicidal if they knew their true situation. With this in mind, *The Patient's Bill of Rights* states:

> When it is not medically advisable to give such information to the patient, the information should be made available to an appropriate person in his or her behalf.

27

DISCUSSION

Although well-intentioned, this statement is unsatisfactory and incomplete. It seems to indicate that when health care professionals feel that harm might result if the patient knows the truth, they fulfill their obligation by telling some friend or family member about the patient's condition and prognosis. The statement does not indicate, however, what the family member or the friend is supposed to do once the information has been communicated. In order to ensure proper respect for the patient, another dimension of the situation must be explored.

Even though the medical personnel might fear untoward results if patients are informed of their true condition, it does not mean that patients should never be told the truth. Indeed, health care professionals should remember in these cases the words of Eric Cassell, M.D.:

> The depression in patients that commonly occurs after the diagnosis of a fatal disease seems to stem in part from the conspiracy of silence. The physician can be a great help by simply making it clear to the patient that he is available for open and direct communication.[1]

Interviews with ill or dying patients reveal that they do not wish to be kept continually in doubt about their condition; however, they do not want it revealed to them in an abrupt or brutal manner. According to Howard Brody, M.D.:

> A decision to reveal a grave prognosis, which may be "ethical" in itself, may become "unethical" if the physician tells the patient bluntly and then withdraws, without offering any emotional support to help the patient resolve his feelings. In fact, the assurance that the physician plans to see it through along with the patient, and that he will always make himself available to offer any comfort possible, may be more important than the bad news itself. In many of the "sour cases" that are offered as justification for withholding the truth, it may well be the absence of this transmission of compassion, rather than the telling of the truth, that produced the unfortunate result.[2]

Because physicians are not always able to convey information concerning serious illness or impending death in a fitting manner, a person trained in the dynamics of accepting sickness and death is useful in the present-day hospital setting. Crisis counseling of this nature is not an arcane art, but, on the other hand, one must be prepared competently in order to perform it well. Well-meaning but untrained people can do more harm than good when trying to help in crises.

CONCLUSION

In summary, it is clear that because of the general public's increased knowledge of psychology and greater regard for the subjective process that accompanies sickness and dying, the ethical question in regard to truth telling has changed. The question should not be "Should we tell?" but rather, "How do we share this information with the patient?"

NOTES

1. Eric Cassell, *The Healer's Art* (Philadelphia: J.B. Lippincott, 1976), 197.
2. Howard Brody, *Ethical Decisions in Medicine* (Boston: Little, Brown & Co., 1976), 40.

9: Confidentiality

From the Hippocratic oath to modern ethical codes, confidentiality has been a concern in health care. The fundamental aim of confidentiality is to protect a person from the revelation of important, sometimes intimate, information that if made public, would damage the person's reputation. Confidentiality is a concern for lawyers, teachers, and other professionals but, because the medical relationship is especially sensitive, confidentiality in regard to patients' diagnoses and prognoses is especially important. Thus, confidentiality, in an effort to foster trust, excludes unauthorized persons from gaining access to patient information and requires that people who have such information legitimately refrain from communicating it to others.

Numerous examples of the difficulty of protecting confidential information have surfaced. Recently a technician leaked information about a possible bone marrow donor in California to a young man dying of leukemia in Texas. Court battles were waged for two months because of this breach of confidential records stored in a university computer bank. Does a minor have the right to physician consultation and confidentiality without parental involvement when birth control devices are desired? What are the rights of psychiatric patients in relationship to their files? Can third party payers of medical care demand a copy of the patient's medical records before payment is made? In modern technological medicine, how many people actually have access to a patient's records? Siegler, in 1982, related that one patient who underwent an elective cholecystectomy complained about the number of people writing in or examining his chart.[1] A survey estimated that at least seventy-five people need access to provide quality care.

Are the above examples indications that confidentiality can no longer be guaranteed and is therefore a defunct ethical requirement in the medical profession?

PRINCIPLES

Confidentiality in the medical transaction can be crucial to the goals of the physician and the patient. If the patient does not believe that the physician will maintain confidences, he or she may not supply possibly embarrassing or personal information important for good history taking and diagnostic procedures. Likewise, confidentiality is important during the treatment period, since physician-patient interactions depend on trust. This crucial element of trust in the physician-patient relationship could be damaged in the overall concern for a patient's health. A number of relationships are at stake if trust is broken: patient-physician, patient and all other health care providers, the reputation of the physician in the community, and his or her relationship with other patients. Ultimately, privacy, personal autonomy, the decision-making process for physician and patient, the patient's responsibility for his or her own health, and public health values could be threatened.

DISCUSSION

Very often, many people need access to medical records in order to ensure proper care for patients. In health care facilities where there is a team of healers, all must have access to needed information. Groups of subspecialists, attending physicians, medical students, three shifts of nurses, and a variety of auxiliary services—each necessary to care for a patient—must have access to records that chart the patient's progress. Simplistic solutions to the issue of confidentiality should be avoided. It would be dangerous to isolate information into different compartments as if the patient were not a whole person or as if one could cure the person by attending only to the physical or the social or the psychological dimensions of the patient's life. Although many providers may be involved in care, this does not mean that idle curiosity or simple interest is sufficient reason to have access to a patient's chart. This must be kept in mind by the administrative auditors who have some need to examine a chart and by the health care professionals on the floor who are caring for the patient. Better health care through a number of specialists, especially in a university setting, must balance carefully the patient's right to confidentiality and the need for information.

Computerization of medical records also increases the potential for breaches of confidentiality. Although the latest technology may make the storing and retrieving of valuable information more efficient and less cumbersome, the director of medical records must provide a network to protect privacy. Physicians may usually depend on this when they are in an institutional setting, but they should remember that in private practice it is their responsibility to ensure the safety of this information. This may be difficult when a central computer bank is used, especially when not all the users are physicians.

Another issue, which is more controllable, is the self-discipline required by all when dealing with patient information. Where something is said—in the cafeteria, in the hall, in the elevator—can be crucial. It is not ethical to allow indiscriminate conversation that violates any patient's right to confidentiality to take place in and out of health care facilities. This is pertinent with cases used in classrooms, rounds, literature, and other teaching areas. One should be careful to mask the identity of those whose cases are used in order to respect their right to confidentiality.

Confidentiality has its limits. Increased access is the result of modern medicine, as seen above, because quality care is ensured only through a larger number of people having access to a patient's chart. Without greater access, care could be compromised. There are classic cases that limit the responsibility of confidentiality. When the patient threatens suicide, for example, confidentiality must be broken to prevent harm to the patient and to other members of society. Such a threat may even be an indirect plea for help. Similarly, public health laws require a breaking of confidentiality to prevent harm to society or to innocent third parties. Such is the case with suspected child abuse, contagious disease, or persons that threaten the life of other members of society.

CONCLUSION

Confidentiality is meant to protect persons and the relationships that they have with health care providers; to ensure trust and patient autonomy, and to provide security as health care is given. Modern technological medicine poses a new challenge to older concepts of confidentiality narrowly inscribed in the one-on-one model of health care. Nonetheless, the values that confidentiality was supposed to foster still exist, and their protection must be reexamined in contemporary settings so that the patient's health may continue to be served.

NOTE

1. Mark Siegler, "Medical Consultation in the Context of the physician patient relationship" in *Responsibility in Health Care* (Boston: Reidel, 1982), 141–162.

10: Medicine: Not an Exact Science

Across the United States, compensation is sought for injuries suffered in the course of medical care. In an effort to control medical insurance rates, to limit the size of awards from injuries, and to improve the quality of medical practice, California and other states have revised the laws regarding damages resulting from medical care and regarding certification of physicians. Although some action is needed to limit the extent of the "malpractice mess," many of the solutions apparently are based on a false notion of medicine and health care. To provide some light in this heated discussion, a more accurate notion of medicine and medical judgments seems necessary.

PRINCIPLES

Medicine is not an exact science. An exact science is a body of knowledge that allows one to reach certain conclusions from causes and to apply that knowledge without fear of error. Mathematics is an exact science. Only human error causes defects in mathematical conclusions. Although medicine applies exact sciences—for example, it relies on the sciences of anatomy, biochemistry, or pharmacology—medicine applies knowledge gained from exact sciences to particular people. Medicine aims primarily at the well-being of individual persons. Thus, the specifying element of all knowledge and techniques are used. Medicine is relativized because of this orientation.

Moreover, consider that medicine is concerned with preventing illness and with curing illness. In both cases, medicine cannot formulate specific norms that are certain to apply for all people or express ineluctable diagnoses or prognoses. When prevention of illness or disease is in question, the potential for framing scientific norms or regulations is impossible. Some even maintain that the "science" of preventive medicine has been so overrated as to destroy its worth.[1] One can improve one's well-being to some extent through regimen and discipline and perhaps limit the possibility of contracting certain diseases, but no definite connection exists between life-style and avoiding disease. Although one may never have smoked cigarettes, this is no guarantee that one will never contract lung cancer.

In regard to curing illness, the intrinsic causes of uncertainty and error are even more prevalent and serious. First, individuals are different in their physiological makeup. Thus, medical diagnosis and prognosis are not precise

33

and exact. Through their bodies, human beings may be studied and objectified. From this, general scientific conclusions about health, disease, and etiological agents of disease may be drawn. However, the uniqueness of each human person, which is expressed in the individual's body, cannot be generalized and objectified. The response of each patient to therapy cannot be predicted scientifically. The "art of medicine" is operative when science is applied to the individual. Because the physician assumes responsibility to help the patient strive for health, medicine is a unique form of art because its "work" is a better human being, not merely an improved inanimate object. The uniqueness of each human body is illustrated in all therapies, but most especially in the use of pharmaceutical compounds. Even though drugs are tested for adverse effects through clinical trials before their approval by the Food and Drug Administration, the search for harmful side effects after approval must continue, because pharmacological compounds affect different people in different ways.[2] Penicillin, for example, serves as a forceful antimicrobial agent for most people, but for some people, it triggers a toxic or allergic reaction that may be fatal.

A second factor limiting the certainty of medical judgments is the difficulty in obtaining sufficient empirical evidence to guarantee the certainty of the medical diagnosis. The anatomy of a clinical judgment combines inductive and deductive reasoning and is filled with uncertainties. Symptoms may be similar for several illnesses or diseases. Moreover, even if laboratory tests are used in making a diagnosis, they may vary widely in reliability and accuracy. Thus, even if tests are available and symptoms abound, the diagnosis of an illness is tentative. One conclusion may be more probable than another but far from certain because the "right" information might be unobtainable. In sum, the process of reaching a diagnosis is dialectical, not the result of rigorous scientific reasoning. The potential for misdiagnosis is evidenced by autopsy studies that show the correlation between the cause of death and the clinical diagnosis is far from exact.

Finally, another cause for uncertainty and ambiguity in medical decision making is the value system of the patient. Medicine is primarily concerned with the patient's physiological well-being, but this in turn is directed to the individual's social and spiritual (cognitive-affective) good. In other words, although physiological health is a foundational value of human life, it is not the only value. A patient may have some social or spiritual values that will determine the type of medical treatment he or she chooses to receive. Thus, the "right" physiological therapy for a particular person may not always coincide with the patient's value system. The person suffering from cancer may determine to forgo curative or palliative treatment in order to devote his life savings to his children's education rather than to therapy that may or may not be successful. The importance of the patient's value system and its influence on therapeutic choices is a vital element in medical decision making. Clearly, it is another source of uncertainty in reaching therapeutic conclusions.

DISCUSSION

Why do people believe that physicians are able to make completely accurate diagnoses about illnesses and infallible decisions about healing therapies for various diseases? Why does the general public, especially members of juries, usually presume that "someone has to pay" if a patient suffers an injury in the course of medical care? Pellegrino and Thomasma[3] attribute this prevalent mistaken notion about medicine to Cartesian dualism. Descartes separated the person and the body, seeking mathematical certainty in medicine. As a result, however, he introduced a false dichotomy that presented the human body as a machine, an entity that could be disassembled and repaired like other machines. This concept dehumanizes medicine. Also, one must admit that the medical profession has not sought avidly to dispel the aura of infallibility surrounding it.

Given the intrinsic uncertainty of medical decision making, therefore, plans to evaluate physicians because of their "mistakes" are unsound. Attendance at continuing education programs may be required of physicians, but it is unjust to measure medical acumen by counting "mistakes" or malpractice accusations. Injuries resulting from patient neglect or physician impairment should be declared as such and just compensation offered. For this reason, physician review boards should be composed of consumers as well as professionals. A contract of justice exists between physician and patient, and the physician is held to make restitution if he or she does not fulfill the object of the contract. But the contract's object is not a certain scientific diagnosis or prognosis. Rather, this contract is a dialectical decision founded on scientific knowledge but influenced by the particular physiology of the body; the ambiguity of symptoms, signs, and tests; and the differing value systems of individual persons.

CONCLUSION

Applying the foregoing concepts will not eliminate all problems arising from medical practice. The perspective of the general public, legislators, judges, and juries, however, may be more accurate if they realize (1) medicine is not an exact science, and (2) physicians make judgments that "follow the rules" but that still may be inefficacious. In their diagnoses and prognoses, physicians may be in error through no moral, cognitive, or technological fault of their own.

NOTES

1. Lenn E. Goodman and Madeleine J. Goodman, "Prevention—How Misuse of a Concept Undercuts its Worth." *Hastings Center Report* 16:2, April 1986, 26–27.

2. Gerald Faich, "Adverse Drug-Reaction Monitoring." *New England Journal of Medicine* 314:24, June 12, 1986, 1589–92.

3. Edmund Pellegrino and David Thomasma, *A Philosophical Basis of Medical Practice* (New York: Oxford University Press, 1981), 99.

11 : The Ethical Physician

Self-understanding is the beginning of wisdom, but in order for it to be possible, one must have the benefit of honest reactions from other people. Otherwise, no opportunity exists for objective evaluation and testing of one's subjective thoughts and attitudes.

What is true of individuals is true of a profession as well. Unless the members of a profession receive honest and objective information from people outside the profession, there is little hope for healthy and effective self-understanding. Over the past few years, the profession of medicine has received candid and worthwhile evaluations in regard to its ethical perspectives and standards from scholars outside the profession.[1] Some of these evaluations may be summarized as follows:

1. Most physicians have a "strong sense of vocation" rooted in the original priestly character of medicine and reinforced in American culture by the religious stress on vocation. Yet this religious motivation has been covered over: "The vast growth of science and technology in the four hundred years since Luther has obscured the specifically religious conception of most vocations. The physician seldom speaks of God anymore when discussing his concern for the patient. Yet he still finds satisfaction in measuring up to personal standards."[2]
2. To be effective, physicians maintain they must be motivated and competent and must show concern for the patient. An important component of motivation is physicians' sense of specific competence; that is, they have an important and well-defined service to offer. Much of physicians' personal satisfaction in their work depends on this sense of competence. Most physicians believe they must "care for the whole patient," but only a minority of physicians have a well-developed social conscience.
3. Physicians tend to think pragmatically, so their basic attitude can be characterized thus: "The physician sees himself as a professionally competent person who is in a social position to apply scientific knowledge and to exercise impartial control over the situation in order to achieve the rational goal of curing or helping a sick patient. The patient's part of the job is to trust the doctor and cooperate with him."[3]
4. Furthermore, physicians on the whole do not regard themselves as research scientists, but rather as applied scientists, and they do not clearly experience a dichotomy between the scientific and the humanis-

tic or affective aspects of medicine. Their satisfactions are not theoretical but pragmatic.
5. Physicians take much satisfaction in their professional position as a mark of achievement. This sense of achievement is more important for physicians than monetary rewards, which they do not like to think of as a primary motivation. Moreover, although physicians gain some satisfaction from scientific interest in their work, they gain more from therapeutic results. An important element of satisfaction or dissatisfaction is four.d in the sense of consistency between personal and professional ethics. Thus, physicians do seem to have a common sense of ethical purpose.

DISCUSSION

Some possible ethical biases that medical professionals should be aware of and that medical education should strive to balance if the medical profession is to make good ethical judgments are as follows:

1. On the whole, physicians continue to exhibit the dualistic balance between the scientific and humanistic. The balance is constantly imperiled, however, by the fact that their scientific training is explicit, detailed, and specialized, while their humanistic and moral training is left largely to example and symbols transmitted to them without explicit reflection or criticism. Physicians thus assume that, although science is exact, ethical discourse is vague, subjective, and a matter of opinion. On the one hand, this assumption leads to a kind of moral skepticism; on the other, to a dogmatic rigidity, since no method of dialogue or research for critical consensus is available.
2. Physicians tend "to take a pragmatic view whereby what is most valued is an immediate, practical solution."[4] In ethical matters, this pragmatism may lead physicians to act so that (1) they will not be made to feel guilty if an action is taken against their professional or personal standards; (2) they will not seem inhuman toward the patient; (3) they will not go beyond the limits of the patient to wider social problems; and (4) they may be more concerned about the law than about ethics.
3. Because physicians' motivation is so bound up with their sense of vocation, autonomy, and competence, they resent interference in their own decisions. They believe that only physicians are in the position to make medical-ethical judgments and that they can be relied on to be decent and humane in these decisions. This attitude may lead to deeply felt but simplistic attitudes toward ethical questions.[5]

4. Physicians often resent that so much responsibility is laid on their shoulders. They cannot understand why a wider sociological, religious, psychological, or interrelational view should be their responsibility. Physicians believe such concerns are someone else's business.

CONCLUSION

These attitudes undoubtedly are the result of the medical professional's need to live by a clear motivation, with manageable responsibilities, and to have sufficient freedom for action and personal judgment. If they result in a closed attitude that renders the physician incapable of learning from others or sharing in a team effort to improve ethical treatment of health problems on a social scale, however, they are harmful biases that may lead to gravely mistaken ethical judgment.

NOTES

1. Amasa Ford, *The Doctor's Perspective: Physicians View Their Patients and Their Practice* (Cleveland: Case Western Reserve University Press, 1967), 139ff.

2. Ibid., 140.

3. Ibid., 144.

4. Eliot Freidson, *Profession of Medicine, A Study of the Sociology of Applied Knowledge* (New York: Dodd Mead, 1971), 147.

5. Wendy Carlton, *In Our Professional Opinion* (South Bend: University of Notre Dame Press, 1979), 173.

12: Professionalism: The Essence Is Empathy

The concern for ensuring ethical behavior on the part of health care professionals continues to mount. The U.S. Congress approved regulations that limit the investments in clinics and laboratories by physicians receiving Medicare or Medicaid payments. The American Surgical Association states norms to control promotional activities of members lest they receive undue compensation from medical supply or pharmaceutical companies. Prominent voices in health care comment concerning the erosion of trust that results from entrepreneurial activities of physicians and hospitals. Will the aforementioned admonitions and norms be effective? Not if they stand alone. To create an ethical atmosphere in the corporate culture of health care, a renewed emphasis upon self-fulfillment through service to patients is needed. In a word, a sense of professionalism must be fostered in order to ensure that ethics leaves the realm of theory and becomes characteristic of everyday activities of health care professionals. In this essay we shall consider the meaning of professionalism and its implications for people in health care.

PRINCIPLES

Professionalism requires knowledge, skill, and empathy. The knowledge required to qualify as a professional varies depending upon one's role in the provision of health care. In the past, physicians were considered the only health care professionals, but in the last century, nursing was recognized as a profession as well. In this century, many additional occupations and services in health care have been recognized as professions because of additional knowledge of human physiology and psychology and the skills developed to apply this knowledge. In our day, therefore, several new professionals may be enumerated in the field of health care, for example, physicians assistants, physical therapists, and health care administrators.

Clearly, acquiring the knowledge necessary for professional practice is not accomplished "once and for all." The need to continue learning even after having attained professional status is well recognized. Unfortunately, many health care professionals confine continuing education to their own specialties. While emphasis upon improving scientific knowledge is laudable, some effort to advance in humanistic knowledge is also useful if one is to progress as a professional.

The skills associated with a profession are designed to utilize effectively the knowledge proper to that profession. In the United States, the effort to acquire knowledge and skills simultaneously is highly developed in the health care professions. All health care educational programs feature clinical experience as an integral element.

While knowledge and skill are important, the distinguishing characteristic of any profession is empathy, or the ability "to get inside" the patient or client. Empathy is defined in *Webster* as "the capacity for participation in another's feelings and ideas." Professions are distinguished from trades, crafts, or commercial occupations by reason of the need for empathy. A tradesman or artisan, for example, a plumber or electrician, can perform his or her service even if he or she knows nothing about the person who requested the service. The knowledge and skill of the plumber or electrician ensures that a building will have water and electricity. While the people who utilize the building may benefit from the ready supply of electricity and water, the person installing or repairing the electrical or plumbing equipment need never contact the persons living there. Professionals on the other hand must know their clients intimately in order to accomplish their goals. They help people strive for goods that require cognitive and affective function on the part of the client. Professions are directed toward helping people achieve goods that are fundamental and at the same time esteemed because they are goods that bespeak our humanity. Health, for example, is one of the basic goods of human life. Without health, we have a difficult time performing these actions that are an expression of the fullness of our humanity. Pursuing truth or building community are two endeavors by which one measures one's humanity. Cannot one pursue these goods more effectively if one is healthy?

DISCUSSION

The extent to which empathy is neglected in contemporary society was evidenced in a statement by Tom Peters, coauthor of *In Search of Excellence*, the "bible" for developing effective business organizations. This book emphasizes the importance of values insofar as creating effective business organizations is concerned. But Peters admits that he neglected to stress the need for empathy in developing value-centered people who will develop value-centered organizations. As Peters states: "(Empathy) is a simple notion, but it is the most complex and operationally the most difficult among the principles that all successful institutions observe. There is nothing patronizing or condescending about empathy. It requires a depth of sensitivity that allows one to sense other people's needs, often before they themselves articulate them." Peters concludes: "I am still at a loss as to how to be prescriptive about empathy, but the term will never again be far from my lips."[1]

Even though Peters may be hesitant about being prescriptive in this matter, a few observations about developing empathy are in order. Empathy must be based upon a desire to share one's gifts with other persons. The gifts a professional possesses are knowledge and skill concerning the attainment of an important human good. Being a professional is sometimes described as an altruistic endeavor. In one sense this is true; being a professional is being "for others." But in another sense, being a professional is self-fulfilling because it enables people to "love others as they love themselves."

The second basis for developing empathy is respect, acceptance, and reverence for other people. Before one can cultivate the ability "to participate in another's feelings and ideas," one must have a recognition of the person as "another self." This concept of empathy offers an understanding of why the profession of health care brings out the best in people, and why adequate health care is fundamental to developing a beneficent society.

CONCLUSION

Norms indicating the ethical manner to conduct oneself as a health care professional are useful. But they will not be observed unless individuals have a personal commitment to being professionals in the full sense of the term. Being a professional means more than earning a degree or possessing knowledge and skills. It also requires an ability "to get inside another person."

NOTE

1. Thomas Peters, "In Search of Excellence," *Chicago Tribune,* 6/18/89.

13: Physician Competency: Whose Responsibility?

A few years ago a conference entitled "Physician Competence: Whose Responsibility" was held in Houston, Texas. The fact that three prestigious groups, The AHA, the AMA, and the Association of American Medical Colleges sponsored the conference, indicates that physician competency is a serious issue. Because the conference seemed to focus upon educational methods and federal monitoring of physician activity, there were few useful conclusions. Yet the question is vitally important. What is physician competency and who is responsible for it?

PRINCIPLES

In order to evaluate competency, one must have a clear concept of the purpose of the endeavor to be evaluated. What is the purpose of being a physician? Medicine aims at maintaining human health, and preventing illness and disease. While medicine is directly concerned with the physiological and psychological functions of the human person, it never abstracts from the social and spiritual functions of the person. Rather, it orders the healing and restoration of the physiological and psychological functions to the patient's social and spiritual values. Of course, the competent physician does not make decisions about the patient's social and spiritual values. Those decisions pertain to the person/patient. But insofar as making decisions about the physiological and psychological functions of the patient is concerned, the physician retains a responsibility that is not shared with the patient. The physician is not the slave of the patient, but rather a co-worker, supplying a very important service that enables the patient to strive more adequately for an integral experience of humanity. From this concept of the purpose of medicine an important corollary follows:

> Medicine of its very nature is a moral enterprise. That is, because of the intimate relationship which medicine has to the value area of the patient's life, the social and spiritual function, the physician must be consistently concerned with the morality of his or her actions. Is what I am doing morally good for this person? Clearly the patient or proxy must be heard before the physician reaches a conclusion in this regard.

DISCUSSION

Given this short exposition of the purpose of medicine, the question is: who is responsible for developing the competencies that will enable the physician to perform aptly the profession of medicine. First and foremost, the physician himself or herself is responsible. Being a professional is different from being a technician. A technician can be trained and tested to perform a mechanical task. Teaching a person to be a plumber or an electrician involves a definite body of information and a definite set of procedures to apply the information. Moreover, the testing of the competency of a plumber or electrician is rather easy; does the faucet work, does the light go on? Insofar as a profession such as medicine is concerned however, the preparation and evaluation is much more complex. There is a definite body of knowledge concerning health, disease and illness that must be acquired by the physician but the application of this knowledge will vary from patient to patient. Even if the knowledge is applied accurately, there is no guarantee that the technical results will be successful; no one lives forever! Moreover, the competent physician will guarantee that the social and spiritual values of the patient are respected and will govern the application of the knowledge proper to the medical profession. To put it another way, competency in medicine requires not only knowledge and the ability to apply it, but also the capacity to "get inside" the person being cared for, to know the patient's value system. This ability cannot be taught in the way one is taught plumbing or electricity. Rather, it requires respect for persons, empathy, and compassion—competencies that develop over time and as a result of personal dedication to the purpose of medicine. Clearly, physician competency requires affective as well as intellectual development.

Because no one becomes an accomplished professional as a result of solitary endeavor, the various medical communities are also responsible for developing competency within their members. Achieving and maintaining competency is a lifelong endeavor, and so medical communities are necessary at various stages of professional life. Thus, a medical school will have the responsibility for helping individuals develop the initial view of the medical profession and acquire the basic knowledge necessary for fulfilling the purpose of the profession. But the attitudes and affective dispositions that are an integral part of medical competency should also be initiated in these formative years. This task indicated the importance of effective role models as members of medical faculties engaged in the initial formation of physicians.

The various medical societies within the medical profession, (e.g. internal medicine, surgery, obstetrics/gynecology) should realize that their goal is to help members to develop overall competency, not merely to keep members up to date on latest scientific knowledge or state-of-the-art equipment. The convention agendas of various specialty groups might be analyzed with this more integral responsibility in mind.

If individuals assume responsibility to their own development and if the various medical societies are conscious of their responsibility to enable members to develop the necessary attitudes and knowledge, will evaluation of competency be required? Yes, accountability is an integral factor in developing competency. To date, most evaluations of physician competency has been by physicians. The argument is offered that "lay people don't know enough about medicine to evaluate physicians." Current dissatisfaction with this system however, has led the federal and state governments to intervene, as the aforementioned conference reported. If the purpose of medicine set forth above has merit, it seems that evaluation should be offered by boards composed of both physicians and "lay people." The purpose of medicine is not speculative; it is practical and practical results require an analysis by the people who are effected by those results. Once again, the board composed of physicians and lay people will be interested in evaluating more than speculative knowledge, it will also have the challenge of determining whether the social and spiritual goals of the patient were prominent in the formation of practical medical decisions. No small order, this.

CONCLUSION

While some may challenge the foregoing concept of medical competency and the plan to evaluate it, let us realize that concepts of competency offered in the recent past have proven inadequate, as have the methods utilized to evaluate competency. Otherwise, prestigious societies would not be sponsoring a conference entitled "Physician Competence, Whose Responsibility"?

14: Various Ethical Systems

Why do different people arrive at different solutions to ethical problems in medicine, even if they begin with the same set of facts? Why, for example, do some persons, whether physicians or family members, decide it is an act of mercy to remove artificial nutrition and hydration from a patient in an irreversible coma, whereas others would maintain that the same action would be murder? One reason for disparate ethical decisions is because people use different ethical systems in reaching decisions about right and wrong actions. In this essay, we describe briefly the various systems that people use to reach ethical decisions. Then we evaluate these systems according to their effectiveness in a pluralistic society.

Ethics seeks to determine which actions will contribute to a person's fulfillment or happiness. Ethics presupposes human freedom and human responsibility. When judging which actions to perform, such as whether to gain money by stealing or through work, a person often faces a conflict. One action is good from one point of view: stealing is an easier and often quicker way of obtaining money. The other action, however, is good from another point of view: working enables one to retain personal integrity, respect the rights of others, and avoid the disgrace associated with theft. How do people settle the conflict? Whether they realize it or not, people use a consistent method of ethical decision making when they are faced with such questions. The major systems of ethical decision making are:

1. *Emotivism.* This ethical theory relies mainly on subjective, emotional response. According to this theory, something is right or wrong because "I feel it is right or wrong." In the United States today, this method of ethical reasoning is widespread. Many will defend their own or others' ethical choices as long as the people making decisions are "sincere." This method of decision making leads to exaggerated individualism, as Robert Bellah and others demonstrate in *Habits of the Heart.*[1] Although emotions are an important factor in making good ethical decisions, emotions alone do not offer a sufficient basis for developing a system of shared values in a pluralistic society. Moreover, emotivism does not enable one to measure an action in accord with one's human fulfillment, unless one maintains that emotional satisfaction is the same as human fulfillment.

2. *Legalism.* This ethical system maintains that the law, whether rendered in the written law or in court decisions, determines what is ethical.

46

In health care, this method is often used with a view toward avoiding malpractice litigation. Thus, physicians, hospital administrators, trustees, and their legal advisors often ask, "What will help us avoid malpractice?" rather than, "How do we foster patient benefit?" This method perverts the relationship between ethics and law. Laws should be founded on ethical norms, but the law often falls behind ethical thinking. For example, to assert that artificial hydration or feeding cannot be removed unless there is a law enabling people to do so, ignores the essential goal of medical care. Thus, laws are helpful if they express sound ethical norms, but laws are not the ultimate norm for ethical choices in a pluralistic society. Too often laws and court decisions are based merely upon legal precedent, or upon political expediency. Thus, they are not always a reliable guide for ethical decision making.

3. *Cultural Relativism.* This ethical method decrees that actions are ethical if they correspond to the customs of a society or a segment of society. Simply because people are accustomed to performing actions, however, does not mean this is an ultimate judge of these actions' ethical worth. Probably the most significant examples of cultural relativism for the health care professions are found in the various codes of ethics used by different associations. For example, the American Medical Association's Code of Ethics approves of some actions that are in themselves unethical and disapproves of others that are not unethical. However, no substantial reasons are given for the decisions offered. Does one have to follow the codes in question to be a good physician? In the past, the codes of ethics for physicians have contained blatant violations of patients' rights, especially in regard to informed consent.[2] Thus, customs and codes are only worthwhile if they are subject to more basic ethical evaluation. Something is not ethical in our pluralistic society simply because "everyone does it."

4. *Fideism.* This method of ethical decision making is based upon religious faith in a church or a person. Although church directives may be helpful and fulfilling for human beings, and although many churches offer worthwhile and reasonable explanations for their teachings, the ultimate motivation for accepting the teaching is religious faith. Thus, directives of churches, even though reasonable, will not be accepted in a pluralistic society by people who do not share the same faith.

5. *Reasoned Analysis.* This method judges ethical issues by reasoning about the effect of the action on the important values of life and the consequences of the action on persons involved. This system seeks to discern whether or not the action and its consequences contribute to human fulfillment and happiness. Reasoned analysis in ethical investigation is difficult and intricate because it means one must seek some

common definitions pertinent to human fulfillment and happiness. It also means one must formulate general norms concerning human functions and human values, and be ready to follow these general norms.

Reasoned analysis in ethical decision making is complicated and intricate, but it has been successful in the health care field because many norms have been accepted in regard to ethical health care. For example, all accept that medical personnel should obtain informed consent before treating patients because this disposes for human fulfillment. Likewise, most accept that access to health care for poor people is a public concern. The many volumes published by the President's Commission for the Study of Ethical Problems in Medicine and Biomedical and Behavioral Research are examples of the effort to approach ethics through reasoned analysis.

Although agreement exists on many major ethical issues in medicine, we do not mean to imply that all ethical issues are near solution. The ethical evaluation of abortion is one area in which consensus has not materialized. We do insist, however, that reaching consensus in our pluralistic society on abortion and other converted ethical issues is not possible unless a process of patient and comprehensive examination of the ethical issues occurs through reasoned analysis. Only through this method can consensus be developed concerning actions that foster or impede human development. And only then will we have the opportunity for consensus in our pluralistic society.

CONCLUSION

A number of books describe in detail the various ethical systems. This brief synopsis presents a general idea of each system and why we often differ on ethical conclusions, even though we may begin with the same set of facts.

The next time you seek to make an ethical judgment or are involved in an ethical debate, analyze the method of decision making that you are using. Realize that some methods are not well-founded because they do not ask the basic questions. Also, realize or recall that for our pluralistic society we need a method of ethical decision making founded on the reasoned analysis of shared values.

NOTES

1. Robert Bellah et al, *Habits of the Heart* (New York: Harper & Row, 1985).
2. Carleton B. Chapman, *Physicians, Law, and Ethics* (New York: New York University Press, 1984).

15: Law, Ethics, and Decision Making

With increasing frequency, difficult health care decisions are being made by judges and the courts. The focus of these cases often involves the availability and use of technologies that have the ability to prolong life without, however, being able to restore health. The fear of legal liability among health care professionals and within institutions too often results in decisional authority being removed from its proper locus, i.e. from patients and their families. Two tragic examples of this recurring phenomenon are the case of the Linares baby in Chicago and the case of Nancy Cruzan. In the former case, physicians who were responsible for the care of Baby Linares refused to respond to the repeated requests by the parents to remove the life-support system that was maintaining the baby's life *even though* the physicians agreed that there was no hope that the baby would recover. Fearing the possibility of a lawsuit, physicians told the parents that the life-support system could only be removed by order of the court. Unable to afford the costs of obtaining such an order, the father removed the baby from the life-support system himself and, holding the hospital staff at bay with a gun, cradled the baby in his arms until he died.

Not quite as dramatic but equally as tragic was the case of Nancy Cruzan who was in a persistent vegetative state for more than five years. The Supreme Court of Missouri refused her family the permission to remove life support that was no longer medically effective. The Supreme Court of the United States stated that the Missouri law was constitutional, but did not settle the ethical issue.

Are judges and the courts the appropriate decision makers in these and other similar cases?

PRINCIPLES

Underlying decision making in medicine and health care is the *principle of informed consent*, which holds that persons have a right to accept or refuse proposed treatment options because persons have a general responsibility for their own health. Thus, when decisional capacity is intact, individuals ought to be allowed to decide for themselves which therapies they will accept and which they will reject. When decisional capacity is lacking, as in the two cases mentioned above, it is generally held that decision-making power shifts to a suitable surrogate(s), in most cases the family. The appropriateness of relying on families in such circumstances is grounded in the confidence we place in family members' ability to make judgments either *as the individual would have themselves were they able* or to make judgments *in the individual's best interests*. Why place such confidence in the family? Because it is the family that knows and loves the individual; it is within the community of the family that individuals receive life and develop, at least, in the case of Nancy Cruzan, values and views about such things as life and death. In cases where such values and views were never formed, as in the Linares case, reliance on the family is based on the belief that families have the best interests of family members at heart. Physicians and other health care professionals, upon entering into the care-giving relationship, commit themselves to provide care in a way that is respectful of and responsive to the patient's own values and goals in life. Those values and goals ought to remain as controlling concerns even when the patient lacks decisional capacity. And in cases where decisional capacity never existed (e.g.,infants) the family's expression of what is in the individual's best interests should be given primary consideration.

DISCUSSION

In neither the Linares nor the Cruzan cases were the families allowed to act as surrogate decision makers for their family member. Fearing legal recriminations, care givers in both instances deferred to the courts for decisions that should have been made by the families with input and advice from care givers. In other words, the decisions were shifted from the ethical to the legal forum.

The shift in focus has two significant consequences. First, the courts, reluctantly drawn into the private forum, impose their values and criteria for decision making in a realm where they are neither adequate nor appropriate. For example, in rendering its decision in the Cruzan case, the Missouri Supreme Court placed its interest in maintaining the authority of the state over the interests of Nancy Cruzan, as expressed by her family, to be free of ineffective and burdensome treatment. In doing so, the Missouri Supreme Court showed little regard for the previously expressed views of Nancy Cruzan and even less regard for the integrity of the family unit. In addition, the Court dealt with issues of law (e.g., the extent of the authority of the guardian) rather than with the ethical issues, which ought to have been of prime concern (i.e., whether ineffective and burdensome treatment can, under certain circumstances, be forgone).

Second, when health care professionals, motivated by fear of legal liability, refer cases such as Linares and Cruzan to the courts they abdicate their ethical responsibilities and fail in the basic commitment that they made upon entering into the care-giving relationship. While the fear of both civil and criminal liability is widespread among health care professionals today, there is little evidence that such fear is well-grounded. The President's Commission and others have concluded that the risk of liability or prosecution in cases involving the removal of life-sustaining therapies is minimal "as long as the decision leading to that result has been made in good faith and according to reasonable professional standards and judgment."[1]

In addition, most civil law actions in questions of the use of life-sustaining therapies are brought before the fact and are often attempts by health care professionals (physicians, administrators and others) to protect themselves by having the courts make the treatment decisions.[2]

CONCLUSION

Health care professionals would do well to consider the relationship of law and ethics as they reflect on their responsibilities to patients *and* to themselves. Both law and ethics imply an obligation to follow norms. The obligation of law is to an external norm, the violation of which may result in material penalty—loss of job, fine, perhaps imprisonment. The obligation of ethics is to an internal norm, often referred to as conscience. Violations in this realm result in a weakening or loss of integrity and appropriate authority. Recourse to the law, as in the cases described above, is often motivated by self-interest while professional observance of ethical norms is generally motivated by concern for the well-being of the patient. It is by maintaining a commitment to the *ethical nature* of medicine and health care that physicians, nurses, and others constitute themselves as true professionals. Without this commitment and a sustained willingness to address the difficult questions raised by life-prolonging technologies, there is a danger that health care professionals will become only technicians, well-educated technicians but technicians none-theless.

NOTES

1. Marshall B. Kapp and Bernard Lo, "Legal Perceptions and Medical Decision Making." *The Milbank Quarterly* 64 (1986): 182.
2. Ibid.

16: Ordinary and Extraordinary Means

When discussing the care of a dying patient, people often use the terms *ordinary* and *extraordinary* means as though they solve all ethical questions. But closer analysis often reveals that the terms do not lead to a clear solution. Are the terms useful or meaningful in ethical discourse? They seem to be, if a few distinctions are kept in mind.

PRINCIPLES

Clearly, physicians and ethicists approach the dying patient with different emphases; the ethicist is more concerned with how the person dies, and the physician is more concerned with how to prolong life. When particular ethical cases are being decided, it seems that there need not be any radical disagreement between physicians and ethicists if three truths are clearly distinguished:

1. Physicians and moralists often use the terms *ordinary means* and *extraordinary means* with different connotations.
2. Although the physician has the expertise and the right to make decisions concerning the usefulness of medical effects of some particular means, the patient (or the patient's family) has the right to determine whether a particular means is ordinary or extraordinary from an ethical point of view.
3. If the means are determined from an ethical point of view to be ordinary, then they must be employed; if determined to be extraordinary, they may or may not be employed, the decision being made by the patient (or the family) in consultation with the physician, but ordinary care should continue.

DISCUSSION

In order to explain these distinctions more clearly, the following thoughts are offered.

Physicians often use the term *ordinary means* to describe an accepted or standard medical procedure. A procedure that is new and untested, still in the experimental stage is called *extraordinary* or heroic. Thus from the physician's point of view, most means could be classified as ordinary or extraordinary without any reference to the patient. From a medical perspective, then, a respirator, tube feeding, or use of an artificial heart have at one time been extraordinary but became ordinary by reason of effectiveness and acceptability.

The ethicist, on the other hand, see these terms in a different light. For the ethicist, ordinary and extraordinary means have no meaning unless the patient's condition is known. For example, one cannot designate a respirator or tube feeding ordinary or extraordinary from an ethical perspective unless the patient's diagnosis and prognosis is known. The ethicist assumes that a person has a need or obligation to prolong human life, but that there are limits to this need or obligation. One obvious limit is that one need not do something useless to prolong life. Thus, if a patient dying of cancer contracts pneumonia, it is generally agreed that one may refuse treatment for pneumonia if life would not be prolonged for a significant time. Hence one need not seek all possible cures for a fatal condition if there is little hope that any of them would be successful.

Another limit to the obligation of prolonging life occurs when the means to prolong life would involve a grave burden to the person insofar as striving for the more important values of life are concerned. For example, classical ethicists maintained that a surgical procedure might be declared extraordinary because of the concomitant burden it might involve. Today we might declare a quadruple amputation extraordinary from an ethical perspective not because of the actual pain of the surgery, but because of the burden that life in this condition might impose on the person.

In maintaining that one is free to make a judgment not to prolong life because a grave burden would result, even though prolonging life is possible, we are affirming that although human life is a great good, it is not the greatest good. This is the practical meaning of the word *burden*: making it difficult for one to attain the purpose of life.

Ethically speaking, then, ordinary means of preserving life are the medicines, treatments, and operations that offer a reasonable hope of benefit for the patient or that can be obtained or used without excessive expense, pain, or burden. Extraordinary means are the medicines, treatments, and operations that cannot be used or obtained without excessive expense, pain, or other burden or that do not offer a reasonable hope of benefit.

Some ethicists maintain that the terms ordinary and extraordinary are inadequate for the decision-making task in ethics. It seems the theoretical difficulties could be eliminated if the first question is not: Is this means ordinary or extraordinary? but, rather: Is there an obligation to prolong life? Thus the patient's condition and value system must first be discerned. If the answer to this latter question is affirmative, then the medical means necessary to prolong life are ordinary means from an ethical perspective. If there is no obligation to prolong life, then only procedures that will keep the patient comfortable are ordinary means and all other means are extraordinary from an ethical perspective.

The practical difficulties in applying the distinction between ordinary and extraordinary means to prolong life will always remain. Determining whether it is time to allow oneself to die, or to allow another to die, will always be a complex decision for a compassionate person. This is especially true if the decision involves discontinuing a means already in use. This difficulty is evidenced excruciatingly in the case of newborns with birth defects. The difficulties do not destroy the use of the distinction, however.

Clearly, the physician is responsible for deciding which therapies are ordinary and which are extraordinary, but who is responsible for deciding this matter from the ethical perspective? The physician must be involved in the decision because the diagnosis and prognosis will depend mainly upon his or her science and skill, but the patient has the ultimate responsibility for making this decision. The patient retains this responsibility not only because he or she has the right to determine which values will be pursued, but because only the patient knows the other circumstances, for example, the pain, expense, or inconvenience involved in a particular therapy, which must be considered in making the ethical decision

CONCLUSION

More difficult problems arise when the patient is incompetent and cannot make the ethical decision. Some would refer all the decisions to the courts, but it seems the courts should be consulted only when a manifest injustice might be inflicted on an incompetent patient. More often, the family or spouse should decide for the incompetent patient for two reasons: (1) they love the patient and will decide what is best for the person; and (2) they know the patient's mind and should be able to request what he or she would want. Physicians and family members should cooperate in the decision-making process, with neither group asserting an adversarial position, but with both groups seeking to make decisions beneficial for the patient.

17: Reforming American Health Care

Bill Clinton was successful in his bid for the presidency in part because he assured the American people that health care reform would be a priority of his administration. Public dissatisfaction with the present health care system is at an all-time high. For while many people acknowledge that American health care is highly sophisticated and technologically advanced, they also recognize the many deficiencies of the system. First, needed services are inaccessible to nearly one-fifth of the American population. Second, health care increases its consumption of the GNP at an unacceptable and unsustainable annual rate. Third, the growing cost of health care threatens the competitiveness and profitability of American business and industry both at home and abroad. Finally, the proclivities of both individual and corporate providers within the system often are pursued at the expense of and harm to persons who are in need of health care services. As with many other proposals for reform, Clinton's approach focuses primarily on measures to control costs hoping that this will ensure appropriate access to the system for all persons. The assumption is that changing the financing mechanism will remedy the growing "crisis" in American health care. But this assumption is mistaken. While some limited positive results may follow from a revamping of the way health care is paid for, the real problems of the American system are its priorities and the values and commitments that support them. As a result, the system frequently fails in its basic task: the promotion of the health and well-being of the individuals and communities it exists to serve. Most significant of the values driving the system are: 1) an extreme form of individualism that routinely prefers individual interests over concerns about the community of persons; 2) an endorsement of profit making as primary motive for providing health care services; 3) an uncritical acceptance of technology as morally neutral and as unambiguously in the service of human goods and goals.

While these values are accepted as appropriately characteristic of the "American spirit," when expressed in matters of health and health care, they foster attitudes and practices that are contrary to the pursuit of health. Under the influence of these values, the health and well-being of persons often is threatened by the kinds of services offered, by the manner in which services are provided, and by the priorities that determine both. If reform of the American health care system is to promote the health and well-being of society and of individual persons within it, two things are required. First, reform

55

efforts must begin by recognizing and challenging the values and commitments that drive the present system. Second, ethically sound reform efforts must be grounded in and guided by an explicit value structure that conforms to human reality rather than by one that shapes reality in ways that deform the human and undermine the community of persons.

UNDERLYING VALUES AND DEVELOPING TRENDS IN AMERICAN HEALTH CARE

From conceptions of health to the principles governing the patient-physician relationship, the commitment to radical individualism has been very influential in shaping the American health care system. This has had a twofold effect. On the one hand, paternalism has been unseated as the paradigm for decision making in health care, giving way to a more participative model of shared decision making. On the other hand, however, the influence of extreme individualism has supported the absolutization of personal autonomy in health care. This tendency has three major consequences. First, interpreting autonomy as an absolute norm tends to undermine the legitimate authority of the physician, frustrating the meaning and appropriate goals of medicine. Second, it dismisses the interests of anyone other than the patient as insignificant in the decision-making process. Both of these effects were obvious in the recently well-publicized case of Helga Wanglie. Third, because of the overemphasis on the absolute right of the autonomous person to determine both present and future care, nonautonomous persons are becoming increasingly vulnerable in our health care system. The tragic cases of Nancy Beth Cruzan and Christine Busalacchi bear this out. Both were rendered incompetent before they gave "clear and convincing evidence" of their autonomous decisions with regard to life-sustaining care. As a result, both became captives of a system that mandated ongoing use of life-sustaining interventions regardless of the fact that the interventions offered no benefit to either one.

Finally, among the most disturbing consequences of the increasing tendency to absolutize autonomy are the recurring proposals to legalize physician-assisted suicide and euthanasia. Proponents of "managed death" argue that the only way to ensure that the individual's right to self-determination can be protected and respected is to legalize the right to choose the method and time of death and to sanction the physician's participation in effecting that outcome.

Influenced by the lure of profit making, American health care increasingly has become commercialized. As a result, altruism often is displaced as the central motive for providing health care services. The activities and practices of the pharmaceutical and hospital supply industries bear this out. While making a profit is necessary, when it becomes the dominant motive a number of negative effects follow. First, health care mistakenly is regarded as a private good or commodity to be made available only to those who can afford to pay for it. Second, when seeking to make a profit in a competitive marketplace, competitive tactics tend to serve the needs of providers rather than those of persons and communities in need. Third, because profit making has been accepted as appropriate motivation, profit potential rather than human need too often determines the availability of services. Fourth, rationing of health care based on the ability to pay is given tacit approval when profit making is deemed an appropriate motive. Finally, when profit becomes the primary reason for providing health care, many health care professionals tend to conduct themselves as if they were engaged in just another business venture. Thus, the meaning of health care as a service or ministry offered in response to human need is lost.

As the technologic prowess of American health care and medicine has increased over the last several decades, the traditional commitment to care for persons in need often is supplanted by an unrelenting search for technologically mediated cure. When cure is possible and can be achieved with a reasonable and manageable amount of burden and distress, it should of course be sought. But too often, technology is employed with little regard for the fact that the person is beyond cure and that the limits associated with human reality have been met. For example, many physicians overtreat terminally ill patients, "even when there is no chance for recovery and death is considered imminent."[1] In such circumstances, persons are harmed not only by the physical assault of technology but, more significantly, by the lack of appropriate preparation for dying and death.

CONCLUSIONS

As these trends have developed, the American health care system has become too costly to sustain. More important, it has become unable to respond appropriately to the health needs of the population it professes to serve. Changing the mechanisms for reimbursement and reconfiguring the marketplace offer little hope of promoting ethical reform unless the values and commitments that drive the present system are rejected and others more fitting to that end are adopted. At a minimum, the following is required. First, there must be explicit recognition that the inherent dignity of every human being demands appropriate regard for basic health needs. Thus, the mistaken notion that health care is a private good distributed according to the ability to pay must be corrected by a suitable regard for health care as a public good provided in response to need. Second, it must be admitted that since the dignity of each individual is worked out in the context of community, concerns about promoting the common good should establish the necessary limits to personal autonomy. In that regard, health care policy should foster responsible steward-ship as the principle to be used to guide decision making at all levels in health care. Third, every effort should be made to eschew profit making as a primary motive for providing health care services. Reform efforts should attempt to regain the notion that health care is a service or ministry rendered in response to authentic human need. In addition, policies that seek to promote appropriate reform should include consideration of ways to foster and maintain the altruistic orientation of the health care professions. Finally, if reform efforts are to have any measure of success in structuring a system that serves the health and well-being of this society, they must recognize that the vulnerable members of the human community deserve special consideration in a reformed system.

NOTE

1. Jane Brody, "Doctors Admit Ignoring Dying Patients' Wishes." *New York Times,* January 14, 1993.

18: More on Health Care Reform: Getting to the Heart of the Matter

This essay is offered in reply to a letter commenting on the previous essay in this collection, *Reforming American Health Care*. A medical student wrote declaring his outrage at the suggestion that health care is a public rather than a private good. He is angered by the proposal that his "time, knowledge and abilities," acquired at great personal effort and expense, should be at the disposal of persons in need of his services rather than for sale to them. He feels misled because upon entering medical school: "I and my money were accepted with no mention of all this 'altruism' and 'public good' stuff." He concluded his comments by arguing that claims made on behalf of goods, rights, and professional virtue have no place in public discourse about issues such as health care reform. Such claims, he argues, are matters of religion and divinely revealed truths meaningful and applicable only to believers.

The sentiments of this student are held by many today. Unfortunately, convictions such as these can impede the efforts of those who seek ethical reform of the health care system. Across the nation politicians, legislators, physicians, and others are consumed by debates about each new proposal offered by the reform team gathered in Washington, DC. Included among the many suggestions for improving the American health care system are creation of a global budget; universal access to a standard health benefits package; realignment of incentives to ensure quality of care; implementation of practice parameters to promote more uniform practice; structuring of local markets to ensure managed and effective price competition; and tort reform to decrease the anxiety of health professionals as they seek to provide health services. The merits of each of these proposals is yet to be determined. However, one thing is evident now; each proposal addresses merely a structural concern or deficiency. Efforts to address more fundamental issues are thwarted by the maneuvering of well-known interest groups that lobby in favor of protecting their own "piece of the action." While reconsidering the superstructure of American health care is important, we must realize that structures serve only ancillary purposes. Health care, however, is a service rendered by one person to another in need. Structural reform, while necessary, is not sufficient to produce ethical reform of the health care system. An ethical outcome will be possible only if the persons who provide health care services within the structures reclaim and recommit themselves to an appropriate understanding of what they are about. In other words, adequate reform will be possible only when we affirm the fact that health care is a public good and therefore a right of all persons. In addition, physicians and other health professionals must rediscover the motives that are at the heart of the healing professions and that are consistent with the nature of the endeavor.

PUBLIC GOODS AND PROFESSIONAL VIRTUE

The proposal that health care is a public rather than private good is not a claim based on specifically religious grounds or divinely revealed truth. Rather, it is an affirmation derived from a simple fact about human reality. There are some goods and values necessary for human life and fulfillment that are beyond the grasp of the individual qua individual. Access to these goods depends on more than mere private enterprise and contract. Such goods meet basic needs in ways that are personally enriching. However, when these goods satisfy individual needs, the life of the community is promoted as well. Thus, while these goods address personal realities, they are primarily public in nature. The goods exist only as an effect of social interaction and cooperation rather than as the product of individual effort or endeavor. A public good, therefore, does not belong to any individual as a product or commodity belongs to its producer. Rather, public goods belong to the community of persons and are dispensed to individual members by persons acting on behalf of both. Therefore, to claim a right to such public goods is to do nothing more than to make a reasonable demand to that which makes the community of persons possible.

Education is a public good. While gaining knowledge may be personally fulfilling, an educated populace is essential if a community is to flourish and thrive. This is particularly true in the complex world of today. Thus, every child in America is ensured access to at least a basic level of education at public expense. Education is considered a fundamental right of the individual, not only because the individual will benefit, but also because the community needs educated members. By providing education for its members, the community is strengthened and unity among the members is fostered.

Society expects the teacher, who acts on behalf of the community by mediating the public good of education to students, to be motivated by something other than merely self-interest or personal gain. The "good" teacher is one who desires to lead students to new levels of understanding because it helps the students. Were the teacher to refuse students the opportunity to learn because they could not pay or because the teacher found them unworthy, the community rightly would be incensed. We hold teachers to this higher standard of motivation because of the nature of the good in question.

Health care, like education, is a public good. Health care and the professions that make it available exist because persons become sick. Illness creates needs that are beyond the competencies of individuals. Thus, persons must turn to the community for assistance in seeking health and responding to illness. The community provides needed services because of a twofold recognition. First, the individual is often unable to address her own health needs adequately. Second, when the individual's health is threatened the community is thereby less healthy as well. When society provides health care services for persons in need both the individual and the community are strengthened and derive benefit.

The primary role of medicine and the other health care professions is to mediate the public good of health care to those in need. Physicians and other professionals act primarily as agents of the society in promoting the health and well-being of the community by strengthening its individual members. The nature of the good in question dictates the motives appropriate to the endeavor. Historically, medicine has recognized this by promoting among physicians a commitment to virtues such as altruism. Thus, both upon entering the profession of medicine and upon embarking on each new relationship with a patient, the physician professes to seek first the good of those in need. In other words, patients' interests have priority over physician self-interest. Society rightly expects its health care professionals to adopt this perspective, and it is with that expectation that society licenses members of the health care professions and gives them the opportunity to practice.

CONCLUSION

The concerns of the medical student that stimulated this response are symptomatic of much of what is wrong in American health care today. Like many in our society, this future physician seems to regard health care as just another commodity to be sold for a price to those who can pay. His displeasure at being reminded that he does not own his skills and talents in the same way that a craftsman does is reflected in the increasing tendency among health care professionals to adopt a business rather than service perspective toward what they do. However, this student should not be faulted. He is the product of a society that has failed consistently over the past several decades to act in accord with reason in regard to health care. The loss of regard for the public nature of the good in question and the growing disdain for the self-effacing virtues demanded of those who distribute this good in society should be recognized for what they are. The present crisis in American health care is the result of failed efforts to hold firm against the incursions of elitism, self-interest and profiteering. The proposal to reclaim what has been lost is not based on any religious commitment nor is it made in response to some divine directive. Rather, it is a proposal to let reason dictate appropriate health care reform. That, of course, is no small task. It demands that those involved in the reform effort have a true appreciation of what health care is and is about. Moreover, it requires that all efforts to maintain the status quo either by focusing exclusively on structural issues or by accommodation to the demands of interest groups be overcome. We owe it to ourselves to demand this. And we owe it to those who, like this medical student, have been misled and confused by our lack of resolve.

Hillary, are you listening?

19: Medical Ethics Requires Accurate Distinctions

A few years ago, Larry McAfee, a young man in Georgia, quadriplegic and permanently dependent upon a ventilator, wished to remove the ventilator because in his judgment the use of it resulted in more burden than benefit. Because death would result indirectly as a result of removing the ventilator, Larry McAfee and his family were forced to go to court to gain legal approval for the proposed removal. In reporting the decision of Judge Edward Johnson, one newspaper stated: "Judge Gives Quadriplegic Permission to Commit Suicide"; another stated: "Judge Rules Quad Free To End His Own Life." The reporting of this case reminds us of the importance of making accurate distinctions when making an ethical analysis. Indeed, much of the disagreement and misunderstanding in regard to ethical decisions often seems to stem from a lack of clear distinctions. This essay will analyze some ethical terms that often generate confusion because they maybe used with different meanings.

1. *Terminal Illness*: This term may signify that a patient will die in the immediate future *even if* life-support therapy is utilized; for example, a patient with cancer in several vital organs will die soon no matter what therapy is employed. Terminal illness may also indicate the presence of a fatal pathology that will cause death in the immediate future *unless* therapy or life support is utilized; for example, a person with renal failure has a terminal illness in this sense, but life may be prolonged through dialysis or a kidney transplant. Many believe that a decision to withhold life support may be made only when a terminal illness is present in the first meaning of this term, that is, when the therapy is useless. Catholic teaching allows therapy to be withheld when the second meaning of the term is verified and the therapy would result in a grave burden for the patient. Judge Johnson used this meaning of "terminal illness" in the McAfee Case.

2. *Quality of Life*: This term is sometimes used to signify the physical or mental disability that impairs a person's function, *but the disability does not endanger the person's life*; for example, a crippled person confined to a bed might be said to have a low quality of life if the term is used with this first meaning. However, the term can also be used to refer to a person whose ability to function is seriously impaired as a result of a serious pathology *and whose life is endangered* as a

result of the pathology; for example, a person who is neurologically impaired because of advanced cancer of the central nervous system.

The confusion arising from the use of this term without proper distinction is monumental. Some state: "Life support should never be withdrawn for 'quality of life' reasons." This is true if the quality of life is used in the first sense. But it is not true if quality of life is used in the second sense. Indeed, even people who denounce quality of life as a criterion for removing life support will admit that life support can be withdrawn if the condition of the patient is hopeless. This is an admission that the "quality of life" in the second sense may be used as a reason for removing life support. In order to avoid the confusion arising from use of this term, Thomas O'Donnell, S.J. introduced the term *quality of function* and suggests that it be substituted when "quality of life" is used in the second sense. This substitution seems to obviate the confusion arising from the unspecified use of "quality of life."

3. *Active and Passive Euthanasia*: Through this distinction, people sometimes convey the notion that active euthanasia (inducing a cause of death) is morally wrong, but passive euthanasia (withholding care with the intention of letting a person die) is morally acceptable. But the intention of killing a person either by inducing the cause of death or by being passive and allowing death to occur is ethically unacceptable. Withholding or removing life support from a person is ethically acceptable only if life support will not benefit the patient and the intention of the care giver is to do something morally good; that is, to cease doing something useless or to avoid inflicting a grave burden upon the patient. As Pius XII pointed out, removing life support with the intention of benefiting the patient even if death is foreseen is an application of the principle of double effect (or indirect voluntary).[1]

4. *Ordinary and Extraordinary Means to Prolong Life*: Although people sometimes use this term as though its meaning were self-evident, this term has both a medical and an ethical connotation. From a *medical perspective*, a therapy is ordinary if it is standard or accepted; for example, clearing the air passages of a newborn infant is ordinary care, medically speaking. From the medical perspective, a means to prolong life is extraordinary if it is innovative, unusual, or unproven; for example, gene splicing to cure thalassemia is extraordinary medical care. From an *ethical perspective*, however, ordinary care signifies medical care that is morally obligatory because it is effective and does not impose a grave burden. Extraordinary care is morally optional because its use is ineffective or does impose a grave burden. From a medical perspective, a therapy or life-support device can be judged ordinary or extraordinary before it is utilized for a particular patient.

But from the ethical perspective, the terms may not be applied unless the medical condition of the patient is known. Moreover, from the ethical perspective a therapy or life-prolonging mechanism may be judged acceptable by one person with a low quality of function, but maybe judged too burdensome by another person with the same low quality of function. Not every quadriplegic would make the same decision as Larry McAfee because the use of the ventilator would not be judged a grave burden by some. Indeed, after encouragement offered by other people with disabilities, Larry McAfee changed his mind about removing the ventilator and is still alive today.

When analyzing the burden resulting from therapy, some people consider only the physiological effects of the therapy, or consider the therapy as though it had ethical import apart from the person to whom it will be applied. Thus some people hold up a gastrostomy tube and a can of Ensure at national meetings and state: "Installing this tube and administering nutrition through the tube would never be a grave burden because this tube and Ensure are not expensive and tube feeding does not inflict serious pain." But Catholic teaching in regard to grave burden maintains that the burden from therapy may affect the psychological, social, and spiritual functions of the person, as well as the physiological. Moreover, assessing the burden of a therapy apart from the wishes of the person to whom it will be applied is the same as buying a suit without knowing the size or color. Finally, some would confine assessment of burden only to the very act utilizing the therapy. But as John Connery, S.J. pointed out when considering the history of Catholic teaching in regard to grave burden: "In assessing any particular means, it made no difference whether the burden to the patient was experienced before, during, or after the treatment."[2]

CONCLUSION

The analysis of the foregoing terms is not intended to answer any specific ethical questions. However, the potential ambiguity of these terms indicates the need for clarification of terms before specific ethical judgments are offered.

NOTES

1. Pope Pius XII, "The Prolongation of Life," (11–24–57). *Issues in Ethical Decision Making*, Gary Atkinson ed. (St. Louis: Pope John XXIII Center, 1976).
2. "Prolonging Life: The Duty and Its Limits," *Catholic Mind*, 10/80, 45.

20: On Playing God

Consider the situation: Health care professionals appear on a radio or TV talk show devoted to questions concerning the treatment of severely debilitated patients. If the proposed ethical solution suggests that a person be allowed to die, someone will object to the solution and say "You are playing God." This phrase is usually uttered with the implied meaning: "Life and death decisions in medical care must be left to God. Human beings have no right to interfere with God's work." Is this a reasonable attitude? Is there any sense in which human beings can and should "play God?" Or should human beings be more cautious, withdrawing from decision making when it becomes obvious that death might unavoidably ensue if another good is chosen? Understanding the concept "on playing God" will help us understand better the mission, nobility, and limits of medicine.

PRINCIPLE

The term *God* implies an all-powerful, wise, and good being whom human beings worship as creator and ruler of the universe (*Webster's Dictionary*). God is the provident director of events and happenings in the universe. Those who do not believe in a personal God might substitute for God the term *Nature*, meaning "a creative and controlling force in the universe" (*Webster's Dictionary*).

Is there any sense in which human beings ought "to play God" or "assume the role of nature?" The glory and challenge of being human is that we are called on "to play God": we are challenged to assist nature by being creative and by controlling our own lives and the happenings of the environment. If we are to fulfill our humanity, we must take an active role in shaping our own destiny, help others fulfill their destiny, and maintain the ecology of the universe. We are created in the image and likeness of God. We have powers from God (Nature)—our intellect and our will—that enable us to take an active and determining role in the decisions affecting our lives and our destinies. We can respect and develop our person and capacities, whether mental or physical, or allow them to deteriorate and atrophy. We can build great societies or allow ourselves to destroy one another through bitterness, envy, and violence. We can respect our environment and preserve it for generations to come, or we can ravage it rapaciously and leave a wasteland for our progeny.

Medical research is an illustrious example of our ability and need "to play God." Medical research seeks to improve human life by eliminating disease and improving our quality of life. Would it be fitting for the medical community to remain passive in the face of the AIDS epidemic and say, "This is God's way of punishing people and we must not interfere." Of course not. Rather, the medical research community, at the behest of all caring people, plays God and tries to eliminate AIDS, thus controlling the future and eventually eliminating one more source of human suffering.

In medical matters, most people realize the need to be responsible for personal health. Realizing that they cannot expect God to send medical care unless they do something about seeking out this help, most people will seek medical help if they are ill. Few people realize, however, that we have the power and responsibility to be creative and controlling in regard to other facets of medical care. By working together, we can provide more adequate health care for all members of our society. Moreover, through mutual cooperation, we can improve our environment and the quality of life in our cities.

Although we have the power to play God, or influence Nature, regarding our personal, social, and ecological responsibilities, we do not have unlimited power. God has unlimited power, but to be human is to be limited. Unfortunately, admitting limitations and shortcomings seems to be difficult for human beings. If we choose one goal, it usually means we must relinquish another. By choosing to avoid physical or mental suffering, one with a fatal pathology may also reject life-prolonging therapy and thus hasten death. We cannot "have it all." "Playing God" in the sense of not admitting limitations leads ultimately to personal unhappiness and social disaster. Thus, we are called on to play God insofar as being creative and planning for the future is concerned. To realize this power responsibly, however, we must recognize our limitations.

DISCUSSION

In medical care, the tendency to ignore subconsciously the limitations of knowledge and technique is prevalent. Some physicians, for example, act as though the death of a patient is a personal defeat. Thus, physicians themselves testify that those who have incurable and terminal disease often are not given the same attention as those who may recover from their illness. Given the limitations of human beings, helping people die well is just as much as part of medical care as healing. Knowing when to cure and when to "simply care" is the epitome of the science and art of medicine.

Admitting limitations for research programs is also difficult. Do those who set policy for research programs stop to say, "We can't do everything: what are the most beneficial things we can do with our limited resources?" Rather, it seems that political economic pressures determine the research agenda. In the United States, medical care and research programs emphasize experimental procedures for the few, such as transplants and artificial organs, whereas more basic programs for the many, such as neonatal care, often are neglected. Medical progress requires that some attention be given to experimental procedures, but are policies on research and practice formulated with a view to social as well as personal medical needs? A neutral observer evaluating U.S. research programs' medical practice might state, "These programs are based on the assumptions that medical care can enable people to live forever and that there are unlimited financial resources."

Besides health care professionals, the general public also often presumes that no limitations exist to health care funding. Many consider it an egregious violation of human rights if a representative of a health care facility, especially a Catholic facility, is forced to say, "I am sorry, we don't have the funds to accept you as a patient." True, health care institutions, especially Catholic ones, by reason of the profession to which they are dedicated, should do as much charity care as possible. Institutions as well as individual persons have limits, however, and it is not a violation of others' rights if facilities acknowledge publicly these limits.

CONCLUSION

Playing God in a worthwhile sense means that we realize we are responsible for the destiny of ourselves, others, and the environment. But it also means that, in fulfilling our responsibilities, we must admit our limitations. Admitting limitations is simply another way of saying that we must pose the relevant ethical questions:

- If we can't do everything, what goods or values are more important than others?
- Which research and therapy programs should receive priority? What must we give up in order to provide more equitable access to health care?

21: Autopsy: Ethical and Religious Considerations

At times people are reluctant to release the body of a loved one for autopsy. Are there good reasons for this reluctance? Is it a violation of propriety, ethics, or religion to release the body of a spouse, parent, or child for medical examination? If not, why the continued reluctance?

PRINCIPLES

When a human being dies, the body is no longer unified by the lifegiving principle or soul by which it is a constituted human being. The cadaver of a person, then, is not a *human* body in the proper sense of the word. Insofar as possible, we should avoid referring to the physical remains of a person as though the person existed *in* a human body or was, so to speak, limited by the human body. Although existing in this life, the human person is a substantial unity of spirit (form) and body (matter), not an accidental juxtaposition of two distinct entities. Although the remains of a human body may resemble the body of a living person, and although this resemblance may be prolonged through embalming, the remains are not a human body, but a mass of organic matter, decomposing into constitutive organic elements.

If the corpse of a human person is not a human body, why are people so concerned about proper care for the remains of the deceased person? Why treat it with the respect and reverence that it usually receives? Respect and reverence are due the remains of a human being because of the value of human life that once informed the now inert mass still bearing the image of the deceased person. In order to mourn and express sorrow for the fact that the person will no longer be present in the same manner as before, certain reverential actions are performed that express the love of the people who remain. Respect for the dead body, then, signifies respect for human life, respect for God, and respect for the person who once subsisted with this now corrupting corpse and who now exists in a different modality. Hence the actions, the rituals that people follow when caring for the body of a deceased person, have a meaning beyond their apparent signification.

Autopsy is the examination of a cadaver after death performed in order to provide greater medical knowledge concerning the cause of death. Historically, the first major impetus for autopsies was provided when Frederick II, emperor of the Holy Roman Empire, instructed physicians studying at Salerno and Naples to spend at least one year in the study of anatomy. Theologians expressed the belief that such dissection of the human cadaver could be done with proper respect for the dead as long as the organs were restored to the body before burial.

In accord with the respect due the remains of a human being, then, in an autopsy no organ should be removed from a corpse nor should the body be dismembered in any way unless there is a sufficient reason to justify such an action. Usually the next of kin or the person to whom the corpse is committed for care has the legal right to determine if organs may be removed from the body and if an autopsy may be performed (*Pierce v. Swan Point, 1872*). The right of the next of kin in regard to caring for the human body is not absolute, however. It may be superseded by statements made by the person while still alive, such as a wish to donate his or her body for scientific study, or by the needs of society, such as when an autopsy might help improve medical knowledge.

Today, the benefit of an autopsy occasionally will be to provide knowledge about a rare or contagious disease. In such cases, autopsies should be performed because the good of the community demands it and because increased medical knowledge is needed. If the next of kin were not willing to approve the autopsy, the court could order that the autopsy be performed. In cases of violent death or unattended death, an autopsy is required by law, no matter what wishes are expressed by the next of kin.

Usually, however, the purpose of an autopsy is not to trace the etiology of a rare disease or to discover unknown or violent causes of death. More frequently, autopsies are performed to help health care professionals achieve a higher level of effectiveness in the care of the living. Autopsies are especially useful for the common good when performed in teaching hospitals. The autopsy rate of a hospital is usually a sign of concern for excellence and offers a gauge of professional integrity and interest in scientific advancement. Through autopsies, the diagnosis and treatment a person received can be evaluated and staff members encouraged to observe a high level of proficiency.

DISCUSSION

From a Christian point of view, the practice of allowing autopsies on one's body for scientific research is acceptable and even to be encouraged if a true need exists. Pope Pius XII, for example, exhibited approval of autopsies when he said:

> The public must be educated. It must be explained with intelligence and respect that to consent explicitly or tacitly to serious damage to the integrity of the corpse in the interest of those who are suffering, is no violation of the reverence due to the dead.[1]

According to the prevailing opinion of Jewish scholars, autopsies can be condoned only when there are indications that the information accruing from them may be of value in saving the life of another individual. Thus, postmortem dissections are indicated when an experimental drug or surgical procedure was used and the autopsy is likely to shed some light on the merits of the treatment. Similarly, when death was caused by contagious disease or genetic disorder, autopsies are warranted for the purpose of instituting prophylactic treatment or helping with genetic counseling. Most rabbinic authorities also permit postmortem dissection for forensic purposes when mandated by law. In all cases where autopsies are indicated, they must be limited to the special areas where relevant information may be obtained. After the examination, all organs must be returned for burial.

The teaching of Islam does not allow for voluntary autopsy because it is considered a desecration of the human person who was associated with the body. If the law requires it, however, then the next of kin may acquiesce to it. Unless some law would be broken or public health endangered, it seems the religious beliefs of people who disapprove of autopsies should be respected. It is worthwhile to point out, however, that one reason why medicine in the Islamic world failed to progress after a promising beginning was due to a lack of clinical information that could have been garnered through autopsies.

Because of what it represents, a corpse should be shown respect and reverence. Such respect and reverence is consistent with autopsies that are designed to promote public health and improve medical knowledge, provided proper respect is shown for the cadavers. When people are faced with a decision concerning autopsy, they should be encouraged to approve such a procedure because of the help that will be offered to others.

NOTE

1. Pope Pius XII, *The Human Body* (Boston: St. Paul Press, 1960), p. 382.

22: Standards for Surrogate Decision Making: Best Interests Or Substitute Judgment

With increasing frequency families and others are faced with choices about treatment options for a patient who, because of incapacity, cannot choose on their own behalf. Such was the case when Bonnie Keiner requested the removal of life support from her mother, Dorothy Longway. Mrs. Longway was irreversibly comatose due to extensive neurologic damage following a series of strokes. Her daughter, Bonnie, petitioned the Court to allow her to make this treatment decision for her mother. In offering its opinion in the case, the Illinois Supreme Court raised the following questions: According to what standard(s) should such surrogate decisions be made? How can Dorothy Longway's interests be furthered appropriately when she herself cannot participate in the decision-making process?

PRINCIPLES

The standards that generally guide decision making for the incompetent person in the health care context have a long legal history. The principles of "substitute judgment" and "best interests" were developed originally to instruct guardians in handling financial and property decisions for the incompetent.[1] Today, these same principles are applied when choices about medical care and therapy must be made for those lacking decisional capacity. And while both standards aim at supporting the basic values underlying informed consent in general, i.e., the welfare of the patient and patient self-determination, there are significant differences owing to the fact of incapacity.

Using the substitute judgment standard as a guide, surrogate decision makers are instructed to choose *as the patient would choose* if he/she were able. Thus, decisions made about treatment options under this standard should further the well-being of the patient in light of the *patient's own understanding* of what constitutes well-being. What this requires, of course, is knowledge of the patient's preferences, values, commitments and concerns. Explicit written statements by the patient himself (e.g., a living will) may seem to be the most reliable source of information regarding treatment preferences. However, life-style, past choices and behaviors, and the kinds and qualities of relationships the person developed can also provide reliable insights into the patient's preferences.

When no evidence exists about the patient's desires, the principle guiding surrogate decision making is that of best interests. Adopting the view of the "reasonable person," the surrogate is directed to choose those options that would most likely contribute to the patient's well-being. This principle aims at objectivity by relying on considerations of "relief of suffering, the preservation or restoration of functioning, and the quality as well as the extent of life sustained"[2] to define the limits of "well-being."

Though these principles become operative at different times according to the circumstances of the patient, both are oriented toward promoting the good and well-being of the patient in question.

DISCUSSION

In allowing for the removal of the life-sustaining therapy in the Longway case, the Supreme Court of Illinois accepted the substitute judgment offered by Mrs. Longway's daughter on her behalf. Unlike other courts (e.g., the New York Court of Appeals), the Illinois high court did not require prior explicit written documentation in order to allow a substitute judgment decision. Rather, the Court recognized that the life goals, values, and preferences of Mrs. Longway could be the controlling factors in the present treatment decision even though Mrs. Longway was unable to participate actively in the process *because* the decisions were being made by her daughter who loved her and who had a lifetime of experience observing her mother fashion her own life according to those values and goals.

Some courts, however, in attempting to guard against error and the possible intrusion of subjectivity into the surrogate's decision, have not allowed the substitute judgment principle to serve as the standard. Thus, even in cases where family members were willing and able to make substitute judgment decisions for their family member, some were not allowed to do so because the courts did not find that life-style, past conversations about sickness and death, past health care practices, etc., provided clear and convincing evidence of the patient's preferences and values.[3] Because the patient, while competent, did not write down specific directions about the use/nonuse of life-sustaining treatments, the best interests standard was held to be the appropriate guide for decision making.

In something of an aberration, the Missouri Supreme Court in the case of Nancy Beth Cruzan has dismissed both standards for surrogate decision making and has argued that incompetent persons who have not left prior written directives about medical care surrender the right to have decisions made in accord with their own values and preferences. In these circumstances, the Court contends, the state should intervene and determine treatment in light of the state's interests and values.

This opinion of the Missouri Supreme Court undermines the consent process by denying that the values of the patient in question ought to set the parameters within which treatment decisions are made. But what of the other approaches?

Clearly, when little or nothing is known about the patient, the "best interests" standard is the appropriate guide for decision making. When this is the case, every effort should be made to ensure that it is the *patient's* best interests and well-being that are the controlling concerns rather than the surrogate's biases or the health care practitioner's view of what is "best."

However, when the life-style, attitudes, views, and values of the patient in question are known by others, especially by family members, substitute judgment should be the standard applied in making treatment decisions. Written documentation by the patient, although helpful, ought not to be required before this standard is invoked.

CONCLUSION

The goal of all decision making in medicine and health care is to make choices that support and are consistent with the values and preferences of the patient. The fact of incapacity should not negate a lifetime of prior choice. Relying on the substitute judgment standard whenever possible can help to ensure that the patient's personal value system is the controlling concern in important treatment decisions.

NOTES

1. President's Commission for the Study of Ethical Problems in Medicine and Biomedical and Behavioral Research, *Making Health Care Decisions* (Washington, DC: U.S. Government Printing Office, 1982), 177.

2. Ibid., 180.

3. In re O'Connor (1988). 72 N.Y. 2d 517, N.E. 2d Dist., 534 N.Y.S. 2d 886.

23: Pain: Some Ethical Considerations

Pain is a continual concern of the human community. Indeed, one can envision pain, in one form or another, as the *raison d'etre* of all professions. Pain may arise from many sources: spiritual, social, emotional, or physiological. For health care professionals, pain is described as "an unpleasant sensory or emotional experience associated with actual or potential tissue damage or described in terms of such damage": (Inst. Assoc. for Study of Pain). At one time, pain was considered an unwanted but necessary by-product of disease and illness. Terminal cancer patients, for example would usually experience severe pain as death approached. In recent years, however, a significant progress has been made in the control of pain. Our interest is not in pain as a medical reality, but rather in pain and pain control as they present ethical concerns. Thus, we shall consider the meaning of pain and the ethical response to pain on the part of health care professionals.

THE MEANING OF PAIN

For the most part, health care professionals and patients alike avoid the question: Why pain? But a few considerations garnered from the wisdom of experience and religious tradition may help to put pain in better perspective. The term pain is derived from the Latin term *poena,* which means penalty. Unfortunately, as the book of Job attests, many people take the term *poena* literally and consider illness, disease, and the pain that accompanies them as a penalty for evil behavior. Thus pain becomes for many people a sign of God's displeasure and a punishment for moral faults. But if this were true, only evil persons would suffer and we know that this is not the case. While some religious traditions do trace the presence of evil and pain in the world to a general shortcoming of the whole human race, it is not presented as part of God's original plan nor as a punishment for personal sin.

Having said what pain is not, can we say anything about the meaning of pain? To question the meaning of pain is to question the meaning of all evil, even death. The problem of pain and evil is a Gordian knot that all great religious traditions seek to unravel. How could an all-merciful God allow pain and suffering to exist in the world? How could a loving God allow a young child to suffer from the pain of leukemia; or allow the generous mother of five to die in pain when others, dedicated to their own pleasures, are left untouched? The depth of this question about a loving God and the suffering of the innocent has turned many to agnosticism.

People of faith realize that the questions of pain and suffering will always be a mystery. While people of faith perceive God as provident and loving, they do not know God as God knows himself and so cannot understand why God allows pain and suffering. To say that pain and suffering are a mystery is simply an admission that human beings are dependent upon God and cannot know everything. In the Christian tradition, pain and suffering have been considered as an opportunity for the individual to join his or her suffering to that of Jesus and thus dispose for greater spiritual union with God. Most world religions envision some form of transforming experience through the proper acceptance of pain and suffering.

Because of the effort to transform pain and suffering, Christianity and other world religions have been considered masochistic by critics. However, accepting pain and suffering as a necessary component of human life is not the same as saying that pain and suffering are good or that they are desired by God. Hence, world religions have always considered the conquering and alleviation of pain and suffering as a fundamental responsibility of the human community.

DISCUSSION

What is the ethical response to pain for health care professionals? When a patient is in pain, the health care professional has three ethical responsibilities: (1) to recognize the effect that the pain and suffering of patients will have upon the health care professional; (2) to help the patient transform the pain into a beneficial experience; and (3) to alleviate or remove the pain if possible.

1. A seldom realized phenomenon is the detrimental effect that living with the pain and suffering of patients may have upon health care professionals. Sound understanding of human personality helps us realize that those who live in the presence of pain will be affected by it. If one does not have a beneficial method of dispelling the sorrow of pain and suffering, one becomes insouciant to the suffering of others.

2. While suffering should never be sought for its own sake, at times it cannot be avoided. In these circumstances, it may become a source of spiritual growth. Helping patients use their fear and suffering as a transforming experience requires personal involvement on the part of the health care professionals. Faced with a suffering and dying patient, some health care professionals turn the patient over to the pastoral care team and remain very much in the background. Others see the care of suffering and dying patients as a mutual responsibility with

pastoral care persons. Pediatricians seem to consider it part of their responsibility to help children die in peace.

3. Alleviating and eliminating pain is much more possible today than in the past. As in any other medical procedure, the patient or the proxy for the patient should be consulted in regard to the use of devices to control pain. Many of the methods to relieve pain or alleviate suffering result in reduced awareness or consciousness in the patient. Some people would prefer to experience manageable pain than to lose their power of concentration. Moreover, different persons have different thresholds of pain. Assigning the same therapy for all persons in pain therefore is not an ethical procedure.

4. At times, the need to alleviate pain may require the use of analgesics that indirectly shorten life. In such circumstances, this is an act of mercy designed to relieve pain, not an act of euthanasia designed to kill the person. While the side effect of this act of mercy may be to hasten death, the side effect is unintended. For example, a person removed from a respirator because life-sustaining efforts are unsuccessful will experience dyspnea or severe discomfort. In this case, morphine sulphate or other barbiturate may be administered to alleviate the pain even if death is hastened.[1] Utilizing morphine before determining the actual pain of the patient has been criticized by some as causing death rather than relieving pain. However, patients removed from ventilators follow a predictable pattern involving pain, and this pattern can be reasonably predicted. Thus, using morphine before the patient is removed from the ventilator would seem to be an ethical practice.

NOTE

1. Laurence Scheiderman and Robert Sprag, "Ethical Decisions in Discontinuing Mechanical Ventilation." *NEJM*, vol. 318, Apr. 15, 1988, 984.

24: Suffering and the Need for Compassion

A few years ago, Janet Adkins was diagnosed as being in the early stages of Alzheimer's disease. Less than a year later, she killed herself by using a "suicide machine" invented and offered for use by retired physician, Jack Kevorkian. In defending his involvement in the case, Kevorkian argued that, in light of the circumstances in which Mrs. Adkins found herself, his assistance in her self-induced death was the only appropriate thing to do. Responses from the medical profession, ethicists, and others were swift and fairly uniform in their condemnation of Kevorkian's actions. Citing the Hippocratic oath, which counsels physicians to "neither give a deadly drug to anybody . . . nor to make a suggestion to this effect," critics expressed concern about the erosion of trust in the medical profession that such action could cause. While this is a legitimate concern, it does not get to the heart of the matter.

More to the point, Janet Adkins was suffering, not physically, but psychically. She looked ahead to a life of increasing disability and dependence and found these inconsistent with her view of meaningful life. She went to a physician for help in managing the reality she faced. And the physician did what many others do when presented with this kind of situation: he turned to technology for a "quick fix."

THE LIMITS OF TECHNOLOGY

As a society, we are becoming increasingly and painfully aware that medical "know how" and technology often cannot provide relief for suffering, particularly suffering of this kind. And so the physician, who is accustomed to relying on scientific knowledge and technical expertise to confer power and control over illness, may at times like these experience powerlessness and, as a result, a sense of personal vulnerability. What is called for by way of response is neither the inappropriate application of technology nor the simple quoting of oaths in an attempt to justify passivity, inaction, or withdrawal. Fitting response to suffering demands at least two things of physicians. First, physicians must understand the nature and meaning of suffering as distinct from pain, whether physical, emotional, or spiritual. Second, they must understand that when science and technology have little to offer in response to suffering, the physician still is called upon to be compassionate.

NATURE AND MEANING OF SUFFERING

While suffering may be concomitant with pain, it is not the same as pain. It is a more profound experience wherein the integrity and meaning of the self are threatened.[1] The one who suffers is tormented by fear, not only by the possibility of physical discomfort or loss of life, but of loss of self and self-identity. For example, when a person is told that they have Alzheimer's disease, their first thoughts may be about future isolation from loved ones and friends that can occur because of memory loss or confusion. Often, the suffering person initially retreats into a world of silence in an attempt to "make sense" of the painful reality that threatens, whether that be a disturbing diagnosis, the recent loss of a loved one, or a reversal in the fortunes of life. If the person is to manage the initial threat to self and emerge psychically intact from this period of silence, some ability must be gained in finding words to express, and thereby gain some control over, what is being experienced. The search for words and language has a twofold importance. First, it provides an opportunity for the person to look with a degree of objectivity at the events in the past that threaten the integrity of the self, for example, receiving the diagnosis of Alzheimer's disease. Second, it allows the person to project into the future a new self, one reconstituted in light of the devastating reality that brings on the experience of suffering.

Once the person finds a voice to express the pain and fear associated with the experience, there then exists the possibility for hope in the future, albeit a different future than the one originally anticipated. This is a process of transformation wherein the suffering is not eliminated but is, rather, made manageable and where a new sense of meaning and self-identity can emerge.

As mentioned, technology and scientific expertise offer little in addressing suffering of this kind. As a result, the physician may have a tendency to refer the suffering patient to a counselor, psychiatrist, or chaplain. But the physician's responsibility to the patient does not end at the limits of medicine and technology; nor does the physician's "power" in the healing relationship. Perhaps more than at any other time in the experience of illness, the person who suffers this kind of threat to the self needs to be empowered if healing is to be effected. And empowerment of this kind is possible only through compassionate presence and response to the person who suffers.

THE COMPASSIONATE PHYSICIAN

Unfortunately, the scientific practice of medicine can act as a strong deterrent to compassionate response. Insofar as medicine's focus is pathophysiology, suffering can escape its glance. But more important, medicine's emphasis on deductive science coupled with its suspicion that the subjective element can distract the clinician from scientific data can lead to the "don't get too involved with your patient or you'll burn out" syndrome.

But true compassion demands what the highly deductive and objective approach finds suspect. The compassionate physician is one who is willing to enter into a process with the suffering person and offer help in accepting and moving beyond the reality that poses the destructive threat to the self. This kind of response requires of the physician a degree of identification with the patient that is likely to increase the physician's own vulnerability in the encounter. But "unless the physician has a genuine openness and vulnerability, it is unlikely that the sufferer will experience the encounter as a healing one in the fullest sense."[2]

Movement through the states of suffering from silent fear to hope in a new future is facilitated by the presence of a compassionate other. The physician who is willing to enter this process with a person not only affirms in word and deed who the person is in the present but also affirms and accepts the person who will be in the future.

Of course, no conclusions can be drawn about what Janet Adkins would have done had the physician she went to for help offered her at least the opportunity to search for hope for the future rather than closing off the future with one stroke of technology. One thing is certain. No "salvation" or solutions to the human problems encountered in suffering are offered by narrow reliance on scientific and technological expertise. Empowerment of the one who suffers, and thereby true healing, is effected only by the response of compassionate people.

NOTES

1. Warren Reich, "Speaking of Suffering: A Moral Account of Compassion," *Soundings* 72: 83–104.
2. Howard Brody, M.D. "Compassion, Empathic Curiosity, and the Physician's Power." Paper presented at the Society for Health and Human Values Annual Meeting. Chicago, IL., November 9–11, 1990.

25: Is There a Human Right to Health Care?

Join in a discussion of any social problem, and frequently you will hear the words "human rights". Often, the term is used as an absolute, or as a weapon designed to settle all controversy. The impression is given that if one person has a human right to something, then others are morally obligated to do all in their power to ensure that the person's right is fulfilled, no matter what the nature of that right. Obviously, a few distinctions are in order if the concept of human rights is to contribute to peaceful and productive human relationships. After discussing these distinctions, this essay asks whether health care is a human right and then offers some ethical considerations pertaining to health care as a human right.

PRINCIPLES

Understanding the concept of human rights begins with an understanding of the concept of innate or fundamental goods of human life. Innate or fundamental goods are those goods toward which our instincts and powers are naturally directed. The term human right then is correlative with innate or fundamental good. If something is an innate or fundamental good, then there is a corresponding human right to pursue that good. The Declaration of Independence referred to these innate or fundamental goods as life, liberty and the pursuit of happiness. Philosophers and ethicists have formulated longer lists of fundamental goods. For convenience's sake, all fundamental goods can be reduced to these four: (1) prolonging life; (2) forming human communities; (3) providing for the future of human communities through generation and education of children; and (4) pursuing knowledge or wisdom. Clearly, each innate or fundamental good has other goods closely allied with it. As we seek to prolong life, we realize that food is a necessary good. As we seek to create human communities, we realize that justice is necessary. As we seek to generate and educate children, the necessity of monogamous relationships between mother and father becomes evident. As we seek to acquire knowledge and wisdom, we realize that study and reflection are necessary human goods. Hence, an analysis of fundamental human goods reveals that there are several goods that are so closely allied with the four fundamental human goods that they also are considered to be fundamental or basic goods. Over time, a good that was not fundamental because it was not needed by a majority of people may become a fundamental good. For example, knowledge is a fundamental good because it is necessary for the well-being of individuals and society. Four hundred years ago, most people could acquire the knowledge necessary to lead a good and fulfilled life without going to school. But as life in society became more complex and more knowledge was needed to survive and to thrive, society determined that knowledge could best be communicated through schooling or "education." In time, education or schooling became a basic good, and now society agrees that there is a right to education for all. Hence, the first implication of the term "human right" is that persons have a relationship toward a good that is fundamental, that is, toward a good that is essentially connected with leading a good and fulfilled life. Of course, we also use the word "right" to connote a relationship to a good that is not fundamental, for example, the right to a car or a piece of jewelry, but because these goods do not pertain essentially to human well-being, this type of right is not included in the term "human rights."

Achieving fundamental goods of life is so important for a person's well-being, both as an individual and as a member of community, that people have an obligation to strive assiduously to achieve these goods. In addition, because we are social beings, people should be aided by other members of the community in the pursuit of these fundamental goods. The community aids individuals by preventing others from impeding them in the pursuit of these goods and by supporting people when they need help to pursue these goods. Thus, the term "human right" implies a relationship or natural orientation to a fundamental good, but it also implies:

1. That human beings strive to acquire these goods. The human condition dictates that we will not always be successful in our quest for these basic goods. However our evolution, history, and culture bespeak a moral obligation to strive conscientiously for these goods in order to be a fulfilled member of society.
2. That persons should not be impeded by others in their quest for fundamental goods. We are social beings and will always have limited resources to fulfill the basic needs of all. Justice demands that one person is not impeded by another person as both strive for the goods of life. For this reason society needs laws and courts to ensure equal access to fundamental goods, such as schooling and employment. Thus, the legal system is not a burden but rather a social necessity.
3. That if one cannot strive for a fundamental good through personal efforts, then the community of persons should help in this endeavor. This third implication also flows from our nature as social beings. When describing this third implication, let us realize that striving for the basic goods of life is not "an either-or" situation. Even when we exercise our personal responsibility, we often need the help of others

as we strive to acquire basic goods. Though young persons may be conscientious in seeking knowledge, their success will also depend upon good teachers.

DISCUSSION

What does the foregoing imply insofar as health care is concerned? Is there a human right to health care? Is health care intimately associated with leading a good and fulfilled life? If by health care we mean the assistance of persons and institutions in the health care professions, then it seems health care is so closely related to the good of prolonging life that it is a fundamental good. In times past, many people could seek to prolong life without the help of physicians and nurses or by being cared for in health care institutions. But due to scientific progress in the science and art of medicine, assistance from people and institutions representing the profession of health care is needed in order to strive for health and thus to prolong life. Hence, there is a human right to health care and state and federal governments should institute programs that protect this right.

After acknowledging a personal responsibility of people to strive for health and the access to health care, we must exercise caution. While many people are able to strive for health and health care through their own endeavors, we must not conclude that those who need help are deficient in their exercise of personal responsibility. People do not get sick "because it is their own fault." Moreover, people in the United States who do not have access to health care are seldom responsible for their situation. For the most part, they are victims of an ineffective health care system. Finally, even if some people seem irresponsible in regard to health, the ethics and ethos of health care take account of human weakness. Compassion is an essential quality of the profession of health care and must not be eliminated in the name of personal responsibility.

Society's obligation to prevent others from impeding the quest for health care will not require many positive programs on the part of state and federal governments. However, enabling people to pursue health will require heroic efforts. There must be an effort to control the cost of health care and an effort to provide access to health care for all. Having affirmed the right of the general population to health care and having affirmed the responsibility of the state and federal government to promote programs that will improve the access to health care, several questions remain: Does affirming a right to health care imply that all persons in society should receive the same health care? What is the most fair and effective way to promote funding for the provision of health care: through employee funded insurance programs or through general taxation? Should the provision of health care allow a choice of physicians and health care facilities? Should payment for health care be based upon fee for services, or upon capitation in a health care organization? Simply affirming that there is a human right to health care does not answer all ethical questions in regard to fulfilling the right to health care.

CONCLUSION

There is a human right to health care because health care is required in order to strive for a good and fulfilled human life. As the effort to recognize the right to health care leads to legislation on the part of state and federal governments in the coming years, the need to factor in personal responsibility will be important. But the need to recognize compassion as an essential factor in the provision of health care will be even more important. There is indeed a right to health care for all because it is a basic good. But in making it possible for people to exercise this right and to strive for health, the nature of the health care profession must be respected.

PART TWO

Cases and Conflicts

26: Truth Telling and Alzheimer's Disease

In the early 1960s, studies indicated that a majority of physicians would withhold a diagnosis of terminal cancer from their patients. Physicians cited fears of adverse reactions by patients to information and the destruction of patient hopes as reasons for withholding a diagnosis. By the late 1970s, similar studies demonstrated a radical shift in physician practice. Over 95 percent of doctors now told their patients of the cancer diagnosis. The shift in emphasis in the physician-patient relationship from paternalism to autonomy has led many physicians to disclose the full truth of diagnosis to their patients. Recent literature has examined similar truth-telling questions about Huntington's disease and multiple sclerosis and reached conclusions consistent with that new model of disclosure. Today, a more complicated question arises. What information should be revealed to a patient with an Alzheimer's type disease? Can a case be made for withholding a diagnosis from such a patient? If so, under what conditions can that be done?

PRINCIPLES

Often, people analyze ethical responsibilities on the basis of normative principles such as autonomy, beneficence, confidentiality, and honesty. However, principles may conflict with each other (e.g., autonomy v. nonmaleficence). Thus, a more helpful method of ethical decision making considers the patient's ability to achieve human fulfillment through the integration of physiological, psychological, social, and creative goods.

Understood in this context, the patient has a responsibility to seek health because it is a basic human good. To exercise this responsibility, the patient must have sufficient information to make an informed decision about medical treatment in light of personal values. Because the physician/patient relationship involves mutual responsibilities, the patient and physician have the respective duties to seek out and provide information that will promote responsible treatment choices and life decisions consistent with the patient's effort to seek true human fulfillment. To do this, the physician provides information that: (1) is truthful; (2) is useful; and (3) has the capacity to help patients make reasonable decisions. First and foremost, the information must be truthful because trust remains at the heart of the physician/patient relationship. Deception and failures to disclose information will undermine such a trust. Second, physicians constantly make determinations as to what is useful information, often excluding esoteric medical facts from the sharing process. Ordinarily, useful information is that which a "reasonable" person would desire. However, such a standard for disclosure must be tempered by individual patient needs. The information provided should enable patients to understand adequately their condition and make informed decisions. Third, the information need only provide the capacity to promote patient good. The fact that the information may cause adverse effects (e.g., depression, anxiety, or even suicidal thoughts) should not dissuade the physician from revealing pertinent diagnostic or prognostic information. In fact, physicians frequently offer treatments (surgeries, chemotherapies, etc.) that have potential for adverse effects, yet they are offered if they provide some capacity to help the patient strive after integral human fulfillment. However, if a physician suspects strongly that the information may cause serious and immediate adverse effects, disclosure may be delayed temporarily until appropriate support systems are arranged to help the patient deal with the truth. This involves a particular application of therapeutic privilege wherein less than full disclosure occurs in order to avoid countertherapeutic results. Finally, if the sharing of information has no capacity to help patients strive after their purpose in life, then disclosure is not mandated. This is analogous to a physician not being required to offer a "futile" medical treatment.

Studies support the need for truth telling. Patients with actual diseases or others when presented with a hypothetical diagnosis indicate a desire to know the truth of the diagnosis. Granted, the information may be upsetting for patients at first, but there is no good documentation of the harmful consequences that truth-telling allegedly engenders. Provision of information allows patients to make informed decisions for further treatment and to prepare for the future. In addition, such information relieves patient anxiety caused by a fear of the unknown. Furthermore, disclosure avoids embarrassment when the patient inadvertently discovers withheld information. Finally, by naming a disease, the patient often gains a symbolic control over it.

In sum, patients should be told the truth, not merely for the sake of fulfilling an abstract principle of truth telling—rather the truth is told in the context of concern and compassion in order to promote true human fulfillment. The temporary exception to full disclosure (i.e., the application of therapeutic privilege) must be scrutinized carefully with a view toward creating a situation in which full disclosure ultimately can occur.

DISCUSSION

Like the word "cancer" years ago, today the word "Alzheimer's" strikes terror in the minds of patients and families. Such terror motivated Janet Adkins to commit suicide with the aid of Dr. Kevorkian. Do such cases suggest that information about an Alzheimer's diagnosis be withheld from the patient?

An application of the principles regarding truth-telling outlined above produces a *prima facie* presumption for full disclosure to the Alzheimer's patient. However, additional factors must be considered. First, no cure presently exists for Alzheimer's disease, although there is a growing battery of symptomatic relief. Second, definite diagnosis of the disease occurs only upon histopathologic confirmation after autopsy. Laboratory, clinical, and imaging tests only provide probable diagnosis allowing for possible misdiagnosis. Third, the Alzheimer's patient often lacks capacity to make decisions because they are unable to retain and process information.

Nevertheless, such additional factors do not seem to modify greatly the responsibility to disclose a diagnosis. First, the lack of a cure does not make Alzheimer's unique. Many diseases are incurable yet disclosure is made. The withholding of tragic or terminal diagnoses may subvert the nature of medicine by giving the impression that the sole purpose of medicine is to cure. In reality, sometimes medicine cannot cure. The fact that on rare occasions, patients like Janet Adkins, feeling a sense of hopelessness, choose suicide, should not proscribe truth-telling. Instead, it should motivate health care professionals to provide better comfort and support systems for patients and their care givers. Second, the lack of absolute certainty about diagnosis and prognosis is intrinsic to medicine. Once a doctor is fairly certain about a diagnosis (often evidenced by treatment choices and information shared with the family), patients should be informed. Third, some may argue that by the time a diagnosis is made, the patient is incompetent. However, there are various stages in Alzheimer's disease. In the early stages, patients may retain decisional capacity that results in a mandate for physicians to inform patients so that patients can participate in the decision making process about medical treatment (e.g., experimental drugs) and life in general. Physicians should be sensitive to the real fears and concerns and even denial that patients and families may experience. But, family desires to withhold a diagnosis should not override the physician's primary responsibility to the patient. Compassionate disclosure can aid in ameliorating such concerns. As the ability to diagnose the disease improves clinically and new treatments emerge, doctors will have to become more comfortable with the disclosure of this troubling diagnosis.

As a patient enters the middle stages of the disease process, the capacity to participate in decision making diminishes greatly. Even so, at this stage of the disease, patients may suffer from depression and anxiety that indicate that, although they may not fully understand, patients still "feel" what is going on. Therefore, information about diagnosis and treatment still may have the capacity to affect a patient's life in a beneficial fashion. The physician and family are both instrumental in judging whether such is the case. The extent to which a patient will understand and retain this information is variable, but the effort to include the patient reinforces a fundamental respect for the patient as a person living with a disease process that robs the patient of self-determination. In the final stages of Alzheimer's when a patient has progressed so far in the disease process that no possible meaning or purpose could be derived from any information, then there is no obligation to disclose this "futile" knowledge (futile in the sense that the patient's incapacity makes it unusable). The physician's clinical judgment and the care giver's experience indicate when information no longer provides the capacity for patient benefit.

CONCLUSION

Physicians have a certain latitude and discretion as to how and when to tell patients and families a diagnosis. After the patient and family have a chance to assimilate the information, follow-up visits should be scheduled to allow for questions and concerns to be raised. Families and physicians should resist the temptation to withhold information out of fear of the disease and the effect of disclosure on the patient. Such worries may be projections that may lead to a conspiracy of silence that in turn results in further isolation of the patient. The presumption for disclosure and openness serves to strengthen the physician/patient relationship and ultimately may help to reduce some of the fears associated with diseases like Alzheimer's.

27: Informed Consent in the Neonatal Care Unit

Sheila Clifford weighed 1000 grams when she was born prematurely last summer. Because of her precarious hold on life, she was flown ninety miles to a hospital with a neonatal intensive care unit (NICU) where more thorough and advanced medical therapy was available. Anyone observing the clinical activity upon Sheila's arrival at the NICU would be impressed with the care and concern of the medical team for Sheila. Equally impressive was the care offered by pastoral care personnel and social workers when her parents arrived at the hospital. A sincere effort was made to consider their spiritual and temporal concerns arising from Sheila's condition. However, not much time was spent conferring with the parents about medical management plans. Life-saving procedures were explained, but permission to initiate and continue these procedures was seldom requested. If the definitions of informed consent formulated by some contemporary ethicists were accepted as the norm, the conclusion could be drawn that in neonatal care units, the rights of parents are sometimes violated. According to these ethicists, health care professionals are responsible only to carry out the "autonomous" directives of patients or their proxies. If there would be any disagreement, the directives of the parents should prevail. This essay will consider the issue of caring for infants in the NICU, seeking to explain why the medical team on occasion assumes more responsibility for decision making than do medical teams caring for patients in other settings.

PRINCIPLES

In order to understand the ethical responsibilities of any profession, one must have a clear understanding of the objectives of the profession. Only after this understanding may one proceed to state the ethical norms for the profession. Through fulfilling the ethical norms of a profession, one not only serves the client or patient in need of help from the professional, one also fulfills oneself as a person and develops the skills and virtues proper to the profession.

What are the objectives of the medical personnel of a neonatal care team? Certainly, they provide health care for infants and children at the request of the parents. But they also care for infants as agents of the community or society. Society needs healthy children. Society strives to foster the well-being of children, especially the weaker ones. When infants are born in a

91

debilitated condition, not only their parents but society at large has an interest in ensuring that the ailing infants will become as strong and as healthy as possible. In a very real sense, neonatologists and pediatricians are the delegates of society. They have a direct responsibility to the child that does not stem entirely from the parents. The philosophy behind this delegation and the desire for children to be strong and healthy is not based upon a perverted notion that the child exists for the society. Rather, the delegation results from the assumption that society exists for the individual. Hence, society should support facilities and professions that promote the well-being of individuals, especially the well-being of children.

Maintaining that medical personnel caring for infants and children receive a mandate from society as well as from the parents, does not preempt the responsibilities of parents. Parents are also advocates for their children. But this mandate does indicate that decision making concerning medical therapy for infants and children is a collaborative process. The unifying theme of this collaboration is that both parents and medical team have an ethical responsibility to strive for the overall well-being of the infant or child.

DISCUSSION

Granted the fact the medical personnel, as well as the parents, are advocates for children, what implications follow?

1. Both medical personnel and parents should be concerned with the overall well-being of the child; not only with the possibility of keeping the child alive. Overall well-being is very difficult to judge, especially for infants, but it involves more than mere physiological function. In addition to the function of the infant, medical personnel consider social and economic factors as they assess well-being. There are some cases, especially if severe neurological deprivation is evident, when continuing life support clearly does not result in overall benefit for the infant. However, simply because an infant is physically or mentally impaired does not justify withholding life support. The traditional ethical norms for withholding or withdrawing life support should be utilized, namely, (1) does this therapy impose a severe burden upon the patient, or (2) will this therapy be effective or ineffective insofar as the overall well-being of the patient is concerned.

   Applying these ethical norms to infants is much more difficult than to other persons. The prognosis for infants is always tinged with uncertainty. Every neonatal care professional can cite a case when an infant survived and thrived contrary to professional expectations. Moreover, when judging the future well-being of a disabled infant, we must not underestimate the value of human life. Adults born with genetic or acquired anomalies are vociferous in appealing for life

support for debilitated infants. In making these difficult ethical decisions, it seems that medical personnel caring for infants and children
many times have a greater responsibility toward their patients than do
medical personnel caring for older patients.
2. States and cities should give high priority to the health and well-being
   of their children. Realizing that society has a special interest in the
   health of children, logically leads to the question: Is enough attention
   and funding devoted by society to the health needs of children? Based
   upon every survey and study available, the answer is no. Society
   fulfills its responsibility to some extent in regard to acute care. But
   primary preventative services, follow-up rehabilitation and chronic
   care services are lacking.
3. In our pragmatic society, the notion of protecting and enhancing the
   life of weak and debilitated infants might become unpopular. In the
   near future, prolonging the life of impaired infants will be considered
   by some to be wasteful and ridiculous. There is a growing tendency,
   because of the ability to detect genetic anomalies and other pathologies
   before birth, to recommend the abortion of less than perfect infants.
   But ethically responsible health care professionals march to the beat
   of a different drummer. As Karl Barth, the noted Protestant theologian,
   stated:

No society whether family, village or state, is really strong if it will not
carry its weak and even its weakest members. They belong to it no less
than the strong, and the quiet work of their maintenance and care which
might seem useless on a superficial level, is perhaps more effective than
labor, culture, or productivity in knitting it closely and securely together.
On the other hand, a community which regards and treats its weak members as a hindrance or even proceeds to their extermination is on the
verge of collapse.[1]

CONCLUSION

Sheila survived and is thriving today. Far from signifying a violation of parents
rights to informed consent, the prompt and aggressive medical care given to
Sheila Clifford indicated a collaborative approach to her overall well-being.
This approach is based upon the love parents have for their children, but also
upon the responsibility of health care professionals to foster the future well-
being of society.

NOTE

1. *Church Dogmatics*, Vol. III, n. 4, p. 424.

28: Revisiting Decision Making for the Seriously Ill Newborn

A recent article in the *New York Times* on late term abortions raises renewed concern about the way in which treatment decisions are made for severely compromised newborns. A New York woman learned that the seven month old fetus she was carrying had several severe medical problems that led physicians to question whether the fetus would live. Rather than consider abortion, the mother expressed her desire to carry the pregnancy to term. But when she asked physicians about the possibility of allowing the infant to die after delivery she was told "that was impossible." Moreover, she was informed that if she did continue with the pregnancy she would have to have the baby at a hospital that could provide "the most sophisticated newborn intensive care unit to assure his survival."[1] Based on the earlier information she had been given about the severity of her baby's problems, Mrs. Elfant concluded that use of aggressive interventions to ensure her baby's physiologic survival would not be in his best interests. Since physicians refused even to consider withholding such interventions, Mrs. Elfant felt that she had no other option than to seek and obtain a late-term abortion.

THE PROBLEM

There has been a gradual but decided shift in attitude over the past decade among physicians and others with regard to the care rendered to severely debilitated newborns. This change is evidenced by attempts to save infants with lower and lower gestational ages and weights and those with multiple serious defects. In addition, there is increasing resistance to recognizing appropriate parental rights and responsibilities in decision making about the use or nonuse of aggressive interventions.[2] This attitudinal change is troubling for a number of reasons but particularly because of the potential negative consequences that it can have on the lives and well-being both of infants and their families. Certainly, the good of human life demands that reasonable efforts be made to ensure the survival of newborns suffering from serious medical problems. But physical life is not an absolute value. Maintaining physiologic existence should be aggressively pursued only when doing so offers some reasonable hope that 1) the infant will have some capacity for a meaningful,

94

interactive, and satisfying life, even if to a limited degree; and 2) when such pursuit or the conditions of the life saved do not cause the infant and/or his family serious burden now or in the future.

It is important to consider the impetus for this change in attitude and to critique the behaviors and practices that result by delineating once again the ethical parameters for evaluating the appropriateness of aggressive, life-sustaining interventions including the role that burden assessment plays in this evaluation.

While we realize that most often physicians make treatment decisions based on what they believe is in the best interests of their patients, there appear to be times when factors other than patient well-being become unduly influential in the decision making process. Perhaps the most troubling of these factors, and often the most difficult to overcome, is the fear of legal liability. It is understandable that physicians and other health care providers are concerned about questions of liability given the experiences of the past several years, particularly with regard to care of seriously ill newborns. Recall the adversarial climate that resulted from the intrusions of the federal government into the clinical care setting following the case of "Baby Doe" in 1982. Establishing hot lines that interested parties could call with their concerns about infant neglect and commissioning NICU "swat teams" gave many physicians and other caregivers the distinct impression that they were under suspicion if they did anything less than everything possible. Further, consider how the inclusion of guidelines for treatment of seriously ill newborns in the 1985 DHHS document on Child Abuse and Neglect Prevention contributed to this already threatening practice environment. Narrowly read, the "guidelines" equate withholding and/or removing life sustaining therapies for *any* reasons other than medical futility and cruelty with medical neglect and child abuse. Moreover, because the "guidelines" fail to mention the proper role and importance of burden assessment in overall treatment decisions, many physicians and others wrongly conclude that appropriate (and therefore legally safe) treatment decisions can be made by assessing physiologic parameters alone.

A second obstacle to the appropriate assessment of the use of life-sustaining therapies in the seriously ill newborn is raised by the expanding technologic capacity to maintain life in even the most extreme circumstances. Because these infants represent the most vulnerable and dependent members of the human family, the commitment to give them every opportunity for life is quite understandable. But that commitment should be shaped and sustained by a concern for the present and future integral well-being of the infant rather than by the technologic imperative that too often leads to the conclusion: If we can do something we must do it! When this imperative becomes normative in the application of life sustaining interventions the results for infants and their families can be devastating.

ETHICAL ASSESSMENT OF LIFE-SUSTAINING INTERVENTIONS

Physicians and other care givers must keep concerns about legal liability and the lure of technologic prowess in proper perspective by assessing treatment options according to ethical criteria that maintain the focus of attention on the overall well-being of the infant.

As articulated many times in these essays, the ethical criteria for that assessment require first that the proposed intervention or course of action offers a reasonable hope of being effective. The therapy should serve not only to preserve physiologic life but, in so doing, to promote the integral well-being of the infant, that is, to allow for social and creative function as well. This is, of course, an assessment made more difficult because of the degree of diagnostic and prognostic uncertainty inherent in caring for newborns. But the mere ability to sustain physical life should not preclude the careful and painstaking ethical assessment that commitment to promoting the overall good of the infant demands.

The ethical assessment also demands that proposed interventions be evaluated in terms of the degree of present and/or future burden they involve or impose. Too often, concerns about the influence of "subjectivity" in burden assessment have been so stressed, particularly in the care of seriously ill newborns, that in many instances the real suffering of both infants and parents are discounted as elements essential to the process of ethical assessment. But reason demands at least two things here. First, present and anticipated future physical and emotional demands made on the newborn in attempts to preserve life and correct defects must be given serious consideration. This is particularly true because the newborn experiences life only in the present. The pain involved in a procedure and the lack of maternal nurturing demanded by a treatment modality cannot be mitigated in the infant, as in the adult, by reflection on past pleasures or anticipation of future gains. Thus, parental concerns about the distress the infant might be experiencing must be given adequate consideration because parents speak on behalf of the infant who cannot express these concerns himself. Second, the newborn infant in the NICU is a member of a family. The present and/or anticipated future adversity experienced by the family in doing what they can to promote the well-being of the infant must be taken into account in evaluating the reasonableness of treatment proposals. The fact that a newborn with multiple problems can be "saved" now but left in a very debilitated condition requiring repeated interventions and constant care may demand that a family have abilities, strength, and resources to continue to care for the child in the future that simply are not available to them. While great caution must be exercised in this area of assessment, the parents' legitimate concerns, fears, and conclusions cannot be disregarded or overridden in all circumstances. The future good of the infant will be pursued in the context of the family. Thus, concern about the good of the child should not exclude entirely concern about the continued good and well-being of the family.

CONCLUSION

Mrs. Elfant sought wise counsel and compassionate care for her severely debilitated yet unborn child. She received neither. As a result she felt compelled to terminate her pregnancy through abortion rather than submit her infant to interventions that she felt would be too painful while offering little positive benefit. Somewhere between the physician's conditioned response and Mrs. Elfant's conclusion lies the realm of ethical dialogue and assessment. The good of life demands that the painstaking process of ongoing evaluation take place and that physicians and parents alike remain open to the honest appraisal of effectiveness and burden.

NOTES

1. Gina Kolata, "In Late Abortions, Decisions Are Painful and Options Few." *New York Times,* January 15, 1992.

2. Gina Kolata, "Parents of Tiny Infants Find Care Choices Are Not Theirs." *New York Times,* September 30, 1991.

29: Physician Self-referral: Ethical Issues

Physician self-referral occurs when physicians refer their patients for tests or treatments to medical centers in which the referring physician has at least a partial financial interest. The referring physician does not provide direct patient services at the center in question, but does share in the revenue and profits of the center. Patients may be aware or unaware of the fact that their physicians own the facility to which they have been referred. The propriety of physician self-referral has been questioned by many.[1] In 1991, the Council of Judicial Affairs of the American Medical Association stated that physicians should not practice self-referral. In 1992 however, the House of Delegates of the American Medical Association adopted a more lenient policy that allows physicians to make such referrals if patients are informed of the physicians financial interest and of any alternative facilities for testing or treatment. Later in the year, the House of Delegates reversed itself and joined the Council on Judicial Affairs in condemning physician self-referral. Clearly, physician referral is a contentious topic. This essay will present an ethical evaluation of the issue in the context of reimbursement of physicians for the services that they offer to the general public.

PRINCIPLES

Professional persons render services that promote the common good of the community, or they perform services that promote the private good of individuals. On the one hand, police personnel are committed to maintaining peace and justice in the life of a community. This service benefits all in the community. People in the community receive police protection based upon their needs, not upon their ability to pay. On the other hand, stockbrokers perform a private service. They help people who can pay for the service to make a profit on their investments. Stockbrokers do not help clients invest money unless the clients are able to pay for their services. People who perform a public service related to the common good are compensated by the community for whom they perform the service. In general, activities associated with the common good of the community are not considered as for-profit endeavors. The society limits or eliminates for-profit activity in this section of community life. The police force of a city for example, is not allowed to set up private sources of revenue associated with their police work. If they do, the revenue is considered graft. On the other hand, services performed in the private sector are usually considered to be for-profit endeavors. People who perform a private service are usually compensated in direct relationship to the services rendered. Their compensation may vary greatly depending upon their ability to offer adequately the service in question. If the stockbroker helps people to increase their investments, she makes more money. If she doesn't, she loses customers and her income.

Where do physicians fit in this division of public and private service to the community? Are they involved in a service of the public or private nature? This depends upon the way in which health care is envisioned and managed in a particular country. In most industrialized countries in the world, health care is considered a public service relating to the common good of the country. In these countries, physicians receive a stipend from the community that they serve. Usually, physicians have a definite number of people to care for (a panel) and they are remunerated whether or not the people request medical care. In this system, physicians are considered to be public servants of the community; not private entrepreneurs. In Canada for example, physicians receive a stipend from the federal or provincial government and are not allowed to engage in a for-profit practice. Moreover, in countries in which health care is considered as a service related to the common good, the health care facilities are part of the public system of health care. Physicians and others are not able to own for-profit facilities to which they can direct patients and thus make a profit from these enterprises. In countries where health care is considered a right for all citizens, facilities are either owned by the community or, if privately owned, they are not for-profit enterprises and are integrated into the public system serving the common good of all members of the community. Thus, the concept of for-profit health care is not compatible with the provision of health care as a public service related to the common good.

In the United States, the situation in regard to health care is ambiguous. For some persons, health care is considered a public service pertaining to the common good. For example, the Medicare, Medicaid, and Veterans Health Care programs are of this nature because admittance to these programs is based upon need, not upon ability to pay. Insofar as the greater portion of people in the United States is concerned, however, health care is treated as a private good. Hence, patients need to be able to pay, usually through private insurance, in order to access the system. In the United States, compensation of physicians varies greatly depending upon the type and amount of services rendered. In addition, for-profit health care facilities are welcomed, not merely tolerated and physicians are allowed to act as entrepreneurs. At present, health care in the United States for the most part is a good of the private sector and medical care is looked upon as a commodity in the free market. Compensation for physicians' services is limited only by the free market, as opposed to being limited by the need to provide a public service for society as it is in other countries. Given the manner in which health care is envisioned and managed in the United States, and given the latitude that for-profit corporations have in supplying health care in our country, there does not seem to be anything intrinsically unethical with self-referral by physicians. If for-profit health care facilities are considered an integral part of the health care system in the United States, it seems that physicians have just as much right as anyone else to invest in these facilities.

DISCUSSION

Whether the provision of health care in the United States will be considered a private good in the near future is debatable. The federal government seems intent upon changing the nature of health care in the United States. The two main drawbacks of health care service in the United States, namely continual escalation of cost and lack of access for over 30 million people, are due to treating health care as a private good. But for the time being, most of the health care in the United States is considered a private good. Thus, self-referral on the part of physicians does seem to be in itself an unethical practice. The ethical problems that result from physician self-referral stem from the way in which the centers are conducted, rather than from the fact that they are physician-owned. Recent studies make it clear that self-referral to facilities owned by physicians results in greater costs and more procedures than when patients are referred to independent health care facilities.[2] Moreover, the access to care is often limited by physician-owned facilities. A recent study in Florida for example, showed that no physician-owned centers providing radiation therapy were in inner city neighborhoods or rural areas, while independent facilities, usually in not for-profit hospitals, were located in these areas.

In order to limit unethical practice in physician-owned health care facilities, it seems the following safeguards should be followed: (1) If patients are referred to facilities in which physicians have a financial interest, patients should be informed of this fact. Moreover, as the House of Delegates of the A.M.A. recommended, patients should also be informed of alternative facilities and be allowed to use these facilities, and (2) A board of trustees or directors involving people from the community should be formed to monitor the activities of the physician-owned facility. This board would monitor costs and services in relation to freestanding centers and provide information to the public concerning the activities and profits of the facility. The profession of medicine is undergoing a crisis of confidence insofar as the American public is concerned. This crisis will only be exacerbated if the practices revealed in self-referral centers are allowed to continue. At the heart of effective medicine is trust between physician and patient. There is no surer way to destroy trust than to demonstrate that profit rather than patient well-being is the goal of medical care.

CONCLUSION

Attitudes toward the provision of health care in the United States are changing. Treating health care as a service of the private sector is simply not working. Escalation of costs and lack of access prompt many to call for a recognition of health care as a public service pertaining to the common good. Another factor hastening the transition to a concept of heath care as a public good is the way in which self-referral centers are administrated in the United States.

NOTES

1. A. Sedlow *et al*, "Increased Costs and Rates of Use as a Result of Self-Referral by Physicians," *NEJM* (November 19, 1992) 1502.
2. J.M. Mitchell, and J. N. Sunshine, "Consequences of Physician Ownership of Health Care Facilities," *NEJM* (November 19, 1992), 1497.

30: CPR and DNR Revisited

About sixty years ago, when a person's heart stopped beating and the lungs stopped breathing, the person was declared dead. But through a series of experiments in the 1940s, it was discovered that the heart could be resuscitated through both drugs and electrical stimulation. In 1960, research demonstrated that circulation also could be restored by external cardiac massage. At first, emergency cardiac resuscitation was used mainly in recovery rooms at hospitals and by persons called upon to give emergency medical care, such as lifeguards, police, fire fighters, and ambulance personnel. Later, in the 1970s and '80s, hospitals and many long-term care centers developed policies that mandated resuscitation efforts (CPR) for all patients who suffered cardiac arrest. Experience quickly demonstrated, however, that not all persons suffering cardiac arrest in health care facilities would benefit from CPR. In an effort to designate in advance those patients who would not benefit from CPR, or who did not wish this form of therapy, "Do Not Resuscitate (DNR)" orders were developed in many health care facilities. In spite of the frequent use of CPR and the frequent issuance of DNR orders, there are several ethical issues that continue to occur in hospitals and long-term care facilities in regard to cardiopulmonary resuscitation. In this essay we shall consider some of these issues.

PRINCIPLES

Cardiac arrest occurs at some point in the dying process of every person whatever the underlying cause of death. Hence, the decision whether or not to attempt resuscitation is potentially relevant for all patients. In theory, CPR for cardiac arrest is a multistep process. Usually it includes chest compression, administration of various medications, electrical shocks to restart the heart, placement of a breathing tube (intubation), and placement on a breathing machine (ventilator). In practice however, the medical team conducting CPR will not wait to see if the initial steps are successful before beginning the more aggressive procedures. Thus CPR is usually envisioned as a single therapy aimed at restoring cardiopulmonary function. As such, it may be evaluated ethically as are other life-prolonging therapies. The essential ethical question for its use being: Will it benefit the overall well-being of the patient? Patient well-being is discerned by considering more than the physiological function of the patient. Keeping the patient alive is not the ultimate criterion

102

for ethical medical care. The social and creative function of the patient must also be considered. Specifically, overall patient benefit may be discerned by asking two questions: Does the life-prolonging therapy impose a grave burden upon the patient, and is the therapy ineffective insofar as the overall well-being of the patient is concerned? If either of these questions is answered affirmatively, then there is no ethical imperative to utilize the therapy in question.

DISCUSSION

While the general principles for use of CPR are not difficult to understand, over the years the application of these principles has occasioned several ethical questions. Who should be considered as an apt patient for CPR? For whom should DNR orders be written. Studies demonstrate that severely debilitated patients, for example, those suffering from cancer or sepsis seldom recover cardiopulmonary function after CPR. Even if severely debilitated patients were resuscitated, some patients survived in a persistent vegetative state. Many of those who did recover some degree of cognitive-affective function died of other causes before leaving the hospital. In order to withhold CPR from a patient through a DNR order, it must be determined in advance that attempts at resuscitation would either impose a grave burden upon the patient or be ineffective therapy insofar as the overall well-being of the patient is concerned. When would CPR be considered a grave burden in relation to the benefit it might bring? In this regard, several people mention the broken bones and bruises that may result from the various steps in the resuscitative process. While some physical injury may result from CPR, in most cases it seems that withholding it on the grounds of physical burden would not be reasonable if weighed against the benefit of prolonged life. Perhaps the patient with severe osteoporosis would suffer serious injury from CPR, which would not be offset by the benefits, but it is not immediately evident that others would experience the same burden. When assessing grave burden, other sources of burden besides physiological suffering should be considered. For example, the economic, social, and spiritual effects of the therapy must also be evaluated. The President's Commission on Ethics in Medicine opined that resuscitation efforts usually provide benefits that justify their costs. In itself CPR would not seem to impose a social or spiritual burden upon the patient or the family, unless it could be foreseen that resuscitation would result in a respirator-dependent condition. If this were predicted, it might be considered that living in this condition would be too burdensome and thus request for a DNR order would be in order.

   Would CPR ever be *ineffective* therapy insofar as a patient's well-being is concerned? Would CPR be effective therapy for a person in a persistent vegetative state, or for a person in a seriously demented condition? Would

CPR benefit patients with end stage diseases, such as cancer of the lungs or pancreas, if it would prolong their lives for only a few days? When a determination is made that CPR would be ineffective, it is an admission that this therapy is not conducive to the overall well-being of the patient, either because it is unlikely to benefit the patient (and this should be demonstrated through clinical research) or that it will not benefit the patient even if it does work. Declaring a therapy to be ineffective is an admission that science and medicine are unable to benefit the patient. Declaring a therapy to be ineffective is not the same as saying the therapy will not prolong life.

Who decides whether CPR will be beneficial for the overall well-being of the patient? Who is the person responsible for determining that a DNR order will be issued because CPR will impose a grave burden or be ineffective? For many years, this decision was considered to be the prerogative of the competent patient, or of the proxy, if the patient were incapable of making the health care decisions. But as evidence proving the ineffectiveness of CPR for some patients became more extensive, it was suggested that the attending physician could make this decision unilaterally and not communicate it to the patient or proxy. Thus, the attending physician could determine that CPR was not an apt therapy for certain patients, just as an attending physician can determine that laetrile is not fitting therapy for reversing the growth of cancer cells. In certain circumstances it seems that physicians should make a decision that CPR is not an effective therapy. This is well within the ambit of ethical medicine. But because CPR is considered a standard therapy, this decision should be communicated to the patient or proxy. To write a DNR without communicating this decision to patients or their proxies would seem to violate their moral right to informed consent.

In the everyday practice, the Slow Code, or Hollywood Code is sometimes in evidence. This practice is characterized by "going through the motions," a decision having been made in advance by care givers that the patient will not benefit from CPR, but no one having had the courage to write the DNR order. Similar to this approach is the predetermined decision to utilize only part of the CPR procedures and to withhold electrical shock and intubation if the less aggressive steps do not restore cardiopulmonary function. The many steps of CPR have one goal: to restore cardiopulmonary function. Halfhearted efforts to achieve this goal would seem to be unethical. If the therapy is judged to be effective, it should be utilized in such a way that will ensure its success. Stopping CPR halfway through the process is simply another manner of going through the motions.

CONCLUSION

Does writing a DNR order necessarily imply that the patient should have all life prolonging therapy withdrawn? In general, the answer to this question is no. Each life-prolonging therapy should be judged upon its own merits. But the medical indications that would justify withholding CPR may discourage the use of other therapies. Hence, if a DNR is written for an unconscious patient with end stage disease, it seems an evaluation of all life-prolonging therapy is in order.

31: Ethical Criteria for Removing Life Support

Christine Busalacchi was injured in an automobile accident in 1987. After a series of acute care interventions were unsuccessful, she was diagnosed as being in a persistent vegetative state (p.v.s). Because of the p.v.s. condition, she was unable to eat or swallow. This fatal pathology was circumvented through medically assisted hydration and nutrition. Six years after the accident, when the courts in Missouri finally determined that her medical care should be under the direction of her father, a controversy arose concerning the ethics of removing life support from a person in a persistent vegetative state. Specifically, the question of removing artificial hydration and nutrition from Christine was debated on television, in the press, and among health care personnel. Emotion and pietistic assumptions more often than sound ethical reasoning seemed to prompt most statements concerning Christine's care. In an effort to clarify the proper care of persons in p.v.s., this essay will consider the facts and questions that are relevant for an ethical withdrawal of life support.

PRINCIPLES

When considering the use or removal of life support, the first relevant fact concerns the existence of a fatal pathology. A fatal pathology is an illness, disease, or bodily condition that will cause the death of a person if the effects of the pathology are not circumvented or alleviated. Examples of fatal pathologies are diabetes, cancer, or end stage renal disease. If a fatal pathology is present, the question arises: Should attempts be made to remove, circumvent, or alleviate the pathology through medical therapy? Or should nature be allowed to take its course, thus allowing the person to die of the existing pathology? Should diabetes be circumvented through the use of insulin; should attempts be made to remove the cancer through surgery; or should attempts be made to alleviate the end stage renal disease through hemodialysis? Usually, people wish to combat fatal pathologies by means of medical therapy. They opt for insulin, surgery, or hemodialysis if their lives are threatened. In most cases, there is an ethical conviction as well as a natural intuition to preserve life through medical therapy because it enables one to strive for the important goods of life. What are these important goods? In general, the important goods are preserving life, seeking the truth, loving our families, generating and nurturing future generations, and forming communities with other people. In addition to these goods, each one of us has particular goods that are important to our sense of purpose and well-being.

In some situations however, extending life through medical therapy does not enable the patient to strive for the important goods of life. Or if it does, the therapy imposes a burden that makes striving for the goods of life too difficult. To be more specific, because of the condition of the patient, medical therapy may be either ineffective, thus making it impossible for the person to pursue the important goods of life. Or it may impose an excessive burden, thus making it too difficult for the person to strive for important goods of life. One situation in which medical therapy usually is ineffective occurs when the patient's death is imminent and unavoidable. Hence, a conscious patient, severely debilitated due to pathologies in many organs, may request removal of a respirator because continued existence in this condition will not allow her to pursue any of the goods of life. Moreover, the same decision to remove life support may be made by family members for a loved one, if the hope of recovering consciousness is slight and death is imminent and unavoidable.

Another condition that renders medical therapy ineffective is the persistent vegetative state (p.v.s.). Because of a dysfunctional cerebral cortex, persons in this condition can never again strive for the goods of life that we identify with creative (or spiritual) human function. Their cognitive-affective function is nonexistent and cannot be restored. Thus, they do not have the power to think, love, relate to others, or demonstrate care and compassion, nor can these powers ever be regained. In addition, because of damage to the cerebral cortex, persons in p.v.s. are unable to eat, chew, and swallow. This pathology can be circumvented by means of medically assisted hydration and nutrition. But does use of this medical therapy benefit the patient? Does prolonging physiological function, with the realization that the patient will be unable to strive for most of the important goods of life, mandate continued medical intervention? Simply because a person in p.v.s. may be kept alive does not indicate that the person must be kept alive. Removing life support from persons in p.v.s. is not euthanasia because it neither induces a new cause of death, nor does it imply the intention of killing the patient.

Medical therapy that imposes an excessive burden for a patient may also be discontinued. An excessive burden may affect a patient's ability to strive for a physiological good, a social good, or a spiritual good that is very important to the patient. The excessive burden under consideration need not be directly associated with the therapy but often results from the use of the therapy. Examples of excessive burden that impede the pursuit of more impor-tant human goods occur frequently. A patient with end stage renal disease opts for discontinuing dialysis because he is bedridden and lacks energy to relate to others or care for himself. The father of a family refuses to have surgery because it would involve selling the family home or expending funds designated for the education of children. A Jehovah's Witness refuses a life-prolonging blood transfusion because she believes receiving blood transfusions is a serious sin.

DISCUSSION

The question concerning excessive burden is posed after a decision is made that the therapy is effective. Hence, there are two distinct criteria that come into consideration after the existence of a fatal pathology has been medically ascertained: (1) Is the therapy effective? and (2) If the therapy is effective, does it impose an excessive burden, whether present or future? Both of these criteria require an evaluation of the patient's ability to strive for the goods of life. In some situations even though medical therapy is utilized, it will not enable the person to strive for the goods of life. Such therapy would be ineffective. In some conditions, medical therapy would enable a person to continue striving for the goods of life, but the therapy would also impose burdens that would make striving for the goods of life very difficult. Such therapy would be an excessive burden. Determining whether therapy is ineffective depends more upon objective evidence than does determining excessive burden. Agreement upon the condition that will lead to imminent and unavoidable death or the inability to regain cognitive-affective function may be reached by reason of objective medical diagnosis. But determining excessive burden is much more subjective. Two people may react differently to the burden of prolonged dialysis treatment. Hence, when people are unable to consent for themselves, it is important to have some idea of how they would evaluate the burden, were they able. Finally, because we are social beings, whether patients decide for themselves or through proxies, evaluation of burden must take into consideration the burden placed upon family and community.

One more question is relevant when considering the removal of life support: What is the intention of the people removing the life support? Clearly, actions that are morally good in themselves may be performed with bad intentions. A person may give money to the poor simply to enhance his reputation. Thus, even an external act of charity can be perverted by means of a bad intention. Many people believe that if life support is removed because it is ineffective or because it imposes an excessive burden, the intention of the family or medical team is to cause the death of the patient. If this were the intention of the people removing life support, it would be unethical. But usually, when removing life support because it is ineffective, the intention of family and medical team is to cease doing something futile. When life support is removed because it imposes an excessive burden, the intention is to remove some form of physiological, social, or spiritual burden from the patient. When people remove life support from a loved one because it is ineffective or a serious burden, they often express relief or even joy. Thus, we hear: "Mom has died but she is better off," "Dad's death was a blessing." But what people are expressing through these words is relief and joy that the burden has been removed, not joy and relief that mom or dad is dead. If the ineffective or burdensome therapy could be removed without the ensuing death of mom or dad, then loving children would remove the therapy in a manner that would prolong life. But given the realities of life, when removing life support becomes ethically necessary, the death of the loved one usually follows as an act of nature. It is not desired or intended by the people removing the life support.

CONCLUSION

Four questions summarize the ethical process that should be followed when removing life support.

1. Is a fatal pathology present in the body of the patient?
2. Does resisting the fatal pathology involve effective or ineffective therapy?
3. If the therapy is effective, does the therapy impose an excessive burden?
4. What is the intention of the persons who remove life support?

The ethical process described above is based upon a vision of human life as a quest for goods that fulfill the innate and acquired needs of the person. Human life is a dynamic process of fulfilling interrelated needs through the pursuit of goods. The purpose of medical therapy is to enable a person to fulfill needs by pursuing goods. Often medical therapy accomplishes this goal. But when medical therapy does not enable a person with a fatal pathology to pursue the goods of life, or makes this pursuit too burdensome, then the medical therapy may be withheld or withdrawn, even though death would result.

32: When Life Support Doesn't Help

Judging from the response, many people disagreed with the decision to remove life support from Christine Busalacchi. To strive for understanding in regard to this important ethical issue, it might be helpful to examine the assumptions of people who disagreed with the decision of the Busalacchi family.

Busalacchi was not in a persistent vegetative state. At least six board certified neurologists and neurosurgeons diagnosed Christine's medical condition as persistent vegetative state (p.v.s.). But many people preferred to believe a video shown on several local TV stations. Busalacchi's open-eyed condition, similar to most persons in p.v.s., and her involuntary reflexes were interpreted by many to indicate consciousness. The most interesting part of this assumption is how people will believe a video as opposed to medical diagnosis made after thorough clinical studies and PET scans.

Because Busalacchi could have been kept alive she should have been kept alive. This assumption fails to distinguish between life support that is beneficial for a person and life support that is not beneficial. The ethical responsibility to continue life support ceases if such support does not benefit the patient. When a person is in a p.v.s. condition because the cerebral cortex is damaged and irreversibly dysfunctional, no benefit to the patient results if mere physiological function is prolonged. Does it help persons to continue their physiological function through support of artificial hydration and nutrition if they will never regain the ability to think, love, talk, or relate to other people?

If a family removes life support because it is not beneficial, the family intends to kill the patient. On the contrary, in most cases the family merely wishes to stop doing things that are ineffective or futile. At other times, the family may determine to remove life support because it imposes an excessive burden upon the patient. The intention of family and physicians as they remove life support is not to kill the patient, even though death is foreseen. When life support is removed because it is ineffective or excessively burdensome, death results from the pathology that the life support has been circumventing. Thus the medical examiner of St. Louis indicated that Christine died of the injuries suffered in the automobile accident six years ago.

Removing artificial hydration and nutrition because it is not beneficial results in a painful death for the p.v.s. patient. As the American Academy of Neurology attests, when artificial hydration and nutrition is removed, because the cerebral cortex does not function the person does not feel pain.

There was no burden involved in keeping Busalacchi alive. This assumption yields to the proof of the economic burden incurred by the state and the psychic burden experienced by the family. Family and community burden must be assessed because every person is intimately connected with other people.

The action of the Busalacchi family and the advice given them was contrary to the teaching of the Catholic Church. While Catholic authorities who oppose the withdrawal of artificial hydration and nutrition from p.v.s. patients may be cited, equally authoritative statements may be cited approving of such withdrawal. For example, Bishop Liebrecht of Springfield, MO, and several bishops of Texas have agreed that removing life support from people in p.v.s. is an ethical option. The document of the Bishops Pro-Life Committee does not supersede the opinions of other bishops. One point is beyond dispute: Catholic teaching allows the withdrawal of life support if it is not beneficial for the patient. That is, if the life support is either ineffective or excessively burdensome, it may be withdrawn even if the patient could be kept alive. Effectiveness and burden are determined by patient and/or family reflecting upon the diagnosis and prognosis offered by the medical team.

Finally, allowing the removal of life support when it is not beneficial is very important. If removal is not recognized as ethically acceptable, people will think that their options are limited if therapy is ineffective or severely burdensome. Thus they will start to accept suicide and murder as the only way out of some desperate medical situations.

33: Withholding vs. Withdrawing Treatment: An Ethical Difference?

In 1983, the President's Commission on Ethics in Health Care rejected the principle that stopping (withdrawing) a treatment is morally more serious than not starting (withholding) it.[1] In 1989, the American Academy of Neurology in its commentary on the treatment of patients in a persistent vegetative state avowed: "the view that there is a major medical or ethical distinction between the withholding and withdrawal of medical treatment belies common sense and good medical practice . . . ."[2] Nevertheless, in the world of clinical medicine, confusion remains in regard to this issue, sometimes with tragic consequences. For example, in 1988 Sammy Linares, a six-month-old baby, aspirated a balloon and eventually lapsed into a persistent vegetative state. The father of the child asked that treatment be discontinued and the child be allowed to die. The hospital lawyer insisted that although withholding treatment would be all right, removing treatment constituted killing the child.[3] Eventually the father removed the child from the ventilator at gunpoint. This tragic story suggests that a need exists to review the distinctions between withholding and withdrawing treatment and evaluate if such distinctions have any ethical significance.

PRINCIPLES

Clearly, a physical distinction exists between not starting and discontinuing treatment. One is an action of omission, the other of commission. In many minds, this physical distinction implies an ethical distinction as well. Specifically, some contend that withholding treatment merely allows nature to run its course while withdrawing treatment seems to introduce a new cause of death and kills the patient. The existential emotional and psychological reactions people have to removing treatment reinforce this ethical distinction. Does the ethical distinction between withdrawing and withholding treatment follow from the physical and emotional distinctions? Proper assessment of the moral significance of the action requires an examination of the intentions of the action. When one appropriately withdraws treatment from a patient, one intends to avoid a treatment that has become overly burdensome or now is evaluated to be ineffective. In withholding treatment, similar intentions are involved except one initially assumes that the treatment will be too burdensome or ineffective without a trial course. In both cases one does not intend death but instead chooses no longer to circumvent an existing fatal pathology because therapy no longer benefits the patient. Consequently, on the level of intention, withdrawing and withholding treatment are ethically the same. In this analysis, the underlying intention determines the ethical nature of the action. As the President's Commission explained, the distinction between omission and commission is ethically unimportant albeit emotionally significant. From this viewpoint, withholding treatment can be equally inappropriate as withdrawing it if one in fact has an obligation to supply treatment.

In addition, making an ethical distinction between withholding and withdrawing treatment threatens to compromise patient care in two ways. First, such an ethical distinction implies that once a care giver starts a treatment, it cannot be removed or removal requires greater justification. The paradigmatic case of Nancy Beth Cruzan illustrates the inappropriate patient care that results from such faulty ethical analysis. Of greater concern is that because of the Cruzan scenario, care givers may withhold potentially beneficial care out of fear that once started, treatment could not be removed even if the expected benefit did not result. Second, patient autonomy and the goals of informed consent may be violated as patients receive treatments that they (or their surrogates) may not desire, which can result in burdens (emotional, physical, financial) for the patient, family, and society.

DISCUSSION AND APPLICATIONS

To provide a practical solution to this problem, care givers may offer a treatment on a trial basis with the explicit understanding that if the treatment is ineffective or too burdensome, it can be discontinued. This approach obviates the possibility of wrongly withholding a beneficial treatment out of fear of not being able to remove it, and it promotes legitimate patient autonomy. When a treatment's efficacy is unclear, one requires greater justification to withhold treatment than withdraw it because treatment efficacy cannot be determined until a trial is completed. This trial-basis approach may prevent situations wherein patients (or most likely surrogates) request the indefinite continuation of medically futile treatments.

Nevertheless, despite the reasonableness of this approach, care givers should recognize and anticipate the emotional responses that some people have to withdrawing treatment. The first is the misconception over culpability resulting from withdrawing treatment versus withholding. Second, care givers may be more reluctant to withdraw treatment because of the investment (money, time, energy) that has been made in the patient. However, to continue to offer ineffective treatment will not make previous treatment worthwhile and it can harm the patient's well-being. Third, care givers and family may feel that in withdrawing treatment, they are abandoning or giving up on the patient. Proper and ongoing comfort care can help alleviate such misgivings about abandonment. Finally, fearing the perception by others that some inappropriate criterion precipitated their decision to remove treatment, care givers may make a psychological distinction between withholding and withdrawing treatment. Although care givers should be sensitive to removing treatment for inappropriate reasons, that should not prevent them from withdrawing treatment for sound ethical and medical reasons.

Gail Povar believes that those emotional responses and their associated barriers to good patient care can be reduced further by adhering to four management approaches: clarity, communication, caring, and closure.[4] *Clarity* involves a clear understanding by all parties regarding diagnosis, prognosis, therapeutic goals, and criteria used to judge when to withdraw treatment. Such plans should be reviewed and updated periodically as new information becomes available. *Communication* means that staff members and other care givers communicate important insights, be updated on changes, and be allowed to present concerns or reservations about the progress of treatment. *Caring* suggests that one recognize the emotional impediments to treatment removal and respond in a sensitive way. Such a response involves patient, family, and fellow care givers who may be ambivalent about the removal of treatment. Finally, care givers need *closure* by means of postmortem processing that reviews the caregiving process and allows for ethical reflection and for the grieving process to occur.

The four management approaches will help people understand that there is no essential ethical difference between withholding and withdrawing treatment. The President's Commission points out that there is only one minor exception to this principle.[5] When a care giver offers a patient a treatment, additional expectations may arise regarding the obligation to continue treatment. To withdraw treatment unilaterally is inappropriate because a significant aspect of the management plan is not shared with the patient and an implicit promise to the patient to continue treatment is abrogated. Therefore, care givers should supply patients with information and involve them in a shared decision-making process in order that the patient's best interests are served. Such an approach to sharing information intimates that informed consent in these cases should be flexible and open to change consistent with new medical data.

CONCLUSION

Medicine deals with not only physical problems but also emotional considerations. Sound medical care takes emotional needs and opinions into account. However, sound medical ethics requires a reasoned analysis as well. This study suggests that no ethical distinction exists between withdrawing and withholding treatment. Even though the two "feel" different, such feelings should not interfere with the appropriate ethical and medical care of the patient. Disagreements and confusion over removal of treatment in the clinical setting can be prevented by proper ethical analysis and certain practical approaches to patient care. Such approaches include ongoing comfort care and clear treatment goal setting with the explicit understanding by all parties concerned that treatment can be removed if it is not benefiting the patient.

NOTES

1. President's Commission for the Study of Ethical Problems in Medicine and Biomedical and Behavioral Research, *Deciding to Forgo Life-Sustaining Treatment*, (Washington, DC: U.S. Government Printing Office, 1983), 77.

2. *Neurology* 39 (1989): 126.

3. L. J. Nelson and R. E. Cranford, "Legal Advice, Moral Paralysis and the Death of Samuel Linares," *Law, Medicine and Health Care* 17 (1989): 316.

4. Gail Povar, "Withdrawing and Withholding Therapy: Putting Ethics into Practice," *The Journal of Clinical Ethics* 1 (Spring 1990): 53.

5. *Deciding to Forgo Life-Sustaining Treatment*, 74–75.

34: Enlightened Legislation: Ethical Considerations

On August 2, 1988, six-month-old Sammy Linares swallowed a deflated balloon. The upper airway obstruction resulted in respiratory failure and cardiac arrest. Sammy had no vital signs for about twenty minutes, but a normal cardiac rhythm was established at a neighborhood hospital. Transferred to Presbyterian-St. Luke's Medical Center in Chicago, life-support systems were maintained even after he was diagnosed as being in a persistent vegetative state. When his father, Rudy Linares, requested that his son be removed from life-support, the physicians, acting upon the advice of hospital attorneys, stated that life support could not be removed unless the family obtained a court order justifying such an action. As is well known, on April 26, 1989, Rudy Linares held off health care workers with a handgun, disconnected Sammy from the respirator and held him in his arms until he died. As a result of the legal and ethical furor surrounding the Linares case, the legislature of the state of Illinois recently passed a bill that allows life-support to be withdrawn from incapacitated persons at the request of a surrogate without a court order. In this essay, we shall consider the ethical substratum for the new legislation, as well as some ethical issues that will arise in its implementation.

THE PRINCIPLES

The Health Care Surrogate Act was signed into law on September 26, 1991, by the governor of Illinois. In sum, the new legislation is a response of several medical, legal, and social service organizations to the ethical and legal anomalies demonstrated in the Linares case. While the new law states clearly that both patients with decisional capacity as well as patients without decisional capacity may have life support removed "without judicial involvement of any kind," the major part of the legislation concerns decision making for persons without decisional capacity. We shall concentrate on the sections of the new law devoted to surrogate decision making for persons incapable of making health care decisions for themselves.

One of three conditions must be verified by two physicians before a surrogate may determine that life sustaining treatment should be withheld or withdrawn from an incapacitated person. These conditions are:

  a) *imminent death*, that is, when death is inevitable within a short time, "even if life sustaining treatment would be initiated or continued."

116

b) *permanent unconsciousness*, for which initiating or continuing life support, in light of the patient's medical condition, provides only minimal medical benefit.

c) *incurable or irreversible condition* that imposes severe pain or an inhumane burden, that will ultimately cause the patient's death and for which initiating or continuing life sustaining treatment provides only minimal medical benefit.

The new legislation, which may not be invoked if the patient has an operative living will or durable power of attorney, lists the order in which a surrogate should be recognized, the legal guardian, the spouse and other family members being given priority. Finally, the act exonerates surrogates, physicians, and other heath care providers from legal liability when they follow "with due care" the stipulations of the legislation.

DISCUSSION

Several ethical principles, while not mentioned explicitly in the bill, are the substratum for the legislation. In order to understand the ethical validity of this legislation, these principles should be considered.

a) The ethical responsibility to prolong the life of an incapacitated person ceases when the life support will not benefit the patient. Removing life support when it is no longer beneficial for the patient does not "cause" the patient's death in the moral or ethical sense. The erroneous tendency to equate "causing death" in the ethical sense with the physical removal of life support has been evidenced in many court decisions, especially in the decision of the Missouri Supreme Court in the Cruzan case. The Illinois legislation explicitly states that it is "not intended to condone, authorize or approve mercy killing or assisted suicide," but does not define the difference between the actions approved by the bill and mercy killing. In order to differentiate between mercy killing and allowing to die, the ethical reasoning that allows withholding or withdrawing life support must be understood.

b) Sustaining the physiological function of people when cognitive-affective function cannot be restored is not a benefit for persons in a state of permanent unconsciousness. This common sense conclusion has been denied by those who would allow withdrawal of life support only when death is imminent, i.e., death cannot be avoided even if life support is utilized. Most people who are permanently unconscious are not in danger of imminent death because life support can continue their existence in this debilitated condition indefinitely.

c) Artificial hydration and nutrition is judged by the same ethical norms as all other life-sustaining treatment. Thus, the long debate concerning the ethical evaluation of the use of artificial hydration and nutrition seems to be near a close. The fact that the Catholic Conference of Illinois promoted and supported this legislation is strong evidence, together with approval of durable power of attorney by the Catholic Conferences in other states, that the Catholic tradition in regard to withdrawal of life support allows the same ethical norms to be applied to artificial hydration and nutrition as to other forms of life support.

d) Life support may be withheld or removed if the patient suffers from an incurable or irreversible condition that will ultimately cause death and that imposes severe pain or an inhumane burden. There has been some discussion whether this "condition" applies to persons with ALS, MS or Alzheimer's disease. From the wording of the legislation, it seems that this "condition" does pertain to aforementioned patients because the "severe pain or inhumane burden" is the result of the illness in question and not the result of the treatment for the illness. If a patient with one of these chronic fatal pathologies is declared incapable of medical decision making, it seems the surrogate may ask that life support be withheld or withdrawn because it is of little medical benefit when compared to the "inhumane burden" imposed by the illness on the patient. Ethically speaking, it seems the illness as well as the therapy may be taken into consideration when determining "severe pain or inhumane burden." All would not agree with this conclusion. Undoubtedly, this "condition" of the legislation will cause greater controversy than the other two.

There are two ethical issues involved in the execution of the law that merit explicit consideration. 1) The act requires that the surrogate make his or her decision concerning the use of life support "in consultation with the attending physician." This requirement demonstrates that the physician is much more than a puppet or bystander in the decision-making process. The surrogate cannot possibly make an ethical decision without having some idea of the potential outcome of various therapies. Hence, the ethical responsibility of the physician must be emphasized, as well as the ethical right of the surrogate. 2) It seems that this legislation, as do most legal statements, confuses the primary responsibility of the surrogate. The act states "that the surrogate shall make decisions for the adult patient, conforming as closely as possible to what the patient would have done or intended under the circumstances." Hence, the legislation indicates that the surrogate should make decisions based upon substitute judgment. "Only when the adult patient's wishes are unknown and remain unknown, or if the patient is a minor," may the surrogate make a decision upon the basis of patient's best interest. However, it seems that the primary moral responsibility of the surrogate is to make a decision in the best interest of the patient, no matter what the patient may have said beforehand. While this conclusion is not shared by all ethicists, and by few lawyers, it seems valid for two reasons: (1) the notion that the patient's prior wishes would be able to envision all present circumstances is unrealistic. Substitute judgment is a legal fiction; attributing to it the place of prominence in surrogate decision making leads to contradictions such as those contained in the Cruzan decision of the Missouri Supreme Court; (2) the right and responsibility of family members to act as surrogates for their loved ones is not bestowed by the civil law; rather it follows from our relationship as human beings. True, the civil law may legitimately regulate and facilitate this right of surrogate decision making, but it does not bestow this right. When one makes a health care decision for a loved one, the statements and wishes of the loved one should be considered by the surrogate. But these wishes serve only to indicate the best interest of the patient. They do not serve as an ineluctable mandate that must be followed passively by the surrogate even in the face of evidence that would indicate that substitute judgment is not in the best interest of the patient. In sum, the surrogate, and physician for that matter, is not a robot-like amanuensis of the patient. Rather, the surrogates are, in their own right, called upon to assume the responsibility of making ethical decisions.

CONCLUSION

Moving health care decisions for incapacitated persons out of the courts and into the family forum is highly desirable. For this reason, the Health Care Surrogate Act of Illinois is worthy of commendation. However, application of the new law will require an understanding of the ethical principles that justify the legislation and of some ethical issues that may arise in the implementation of the legislation.

35: Demands for Futile Therapy: When Will We Ever Learn?

A few years ago, a Minnesota judge granted guardianship to Helga Wanglie's husband and directed physicians to comply with Mr. Wanglie's demands for continued life-sustaining care for his wife. Three days later, Mrs. Wanglie died of sepsis while still on full life support in an intensive care unit. In rendering its decision, the court focused primary attention on the locus of decision making. As a result, the significance of the content of the demands being made by Mrs. Wanglie's family were minimized. The fact that the interventions in question had been judged to be medically futile by the physicians caring for Mrs. Wanglie apparently was not a central concern in the court's decision. The ruling in the Wanglie case reflects a growing sentiment that medical decisions about the good of the patient should be reached by consideration of subjective data alone, i.e., the personal values of the patient or family, with little or no reference to any objective information or input provided by the physician. From this perspective, doing what is right and good for persons involves little more than responding to their expressed wants and desires. Thus, the court's decision in the Wanglie case questions the body of knowledge at the heart of medicine. This knowledge does provide objective data for making determinations about human good and how to promote it. The pervasiveness of the attitude reflected in the finding of the court threatens to enervate the profession of medicine and to undermine its basic commitment to human good and well-being.

Mrs. Wanglie's ordeal began when she fractured her hip. Shortly after the surgical repair of the fracture, she began a downhill course that eventually left her persistently vegetative secondary to severe hypoxic encephalopathy. Her physical condition was such that continued physiologic life required full technical support and ongoing intensive care. Although physicians repeatedly informed the family of Mrs. Wanglie's poor prognosis and made it clear that continued medical intervention would do nothing to reverse her neurologic status or improve her overall condition, her husband, daughter, and son insisted that full support be continued. Mr. Wanglie argued that the family's position reflected his wife's earlier statement that "if anything happened to her so that she could not take care of herself, she did not want anything done to shorten or prematurely take her life."[1]

120

In ordering physicians to carry out Mr. Wanglie's demands for continued life-sustaining interventions, the court obviated consideration of the central issue, i.e., the questionable appropriateness of allowing and encouraging patients or their surrogates to demand and receive interventions that are judged to be medically futile. In order to discuss the significance of this case it is necessary to explore the meaning of futility as it relates to medical care and to examine the implications of the court's decision for the future of medical practice.

FUTILITY AND THE PRACTICE OF MEDICINE

"Futile" describes something that is frivolous, trivial, without meaning, or of no consequence. When applied to specific human activity, futility delineates actions that offer no reasonable possibility of accomplishing the goals for which they are performed. In the context of medical practice, futility is used to describe interventions that do not offer a reasonable hope of contributing to the integrated functioning of the person. Medical interventions of the kind used for Mrs. Wanglie (e.g., mechanical ventilator, feeding tube, vasopressor drugs) are not prescribed by the physician solely to address physiologic problems. In seeking the good of the person, the physician renders medical care in hopes of alleviating a physiologic problem *in order to promote the integrated functioning of the whole person* (i.e., integration of the physiologic, psychologic, social, and creative dimensions) thus allowing the person some capacity to pursue life's goals and objectives. While an antibiotic may be successful in treating pneumonia, it would be a futile intervention if used for a person whose overall condition does not allow for integrated functioning, e.g., when the person is in a persistent vegetative state (p.v.s.). In p.v.s. the irreversible loss of function of the cerebral cortex precludes integration of the psychologic, social, and creative dimensions of the person. In p.v.s., while the physiologic level of function can be affected, the person herself cannot pursue human objectives because of the underlying physical condition.[2] On the other hand, while an antibiotic used to treat pneumonia in a person in the terminal stage of cancer cannot reverse the course of the cancer, it may afford the person the opportunity to strive for his objectives in life in a limited way. In the latter case, the conclusion that the intervention is not futile and can be offered to the patient depends on the overall condition of the person and the capacity for some degree of integrated function even in the presence of terminal disease. Note that in the latter example, while the physician makes the determination that the proposed therapy may offer a reasonable hope of benefit for the patient, it is then up to the patient or proxy to accept or refuse the therapy based on his own assessment of potential benefit and associated burden.

Determinations of medical futility are based both on clinical data (e.g., the findings of physical examination, laboratory reports, x-ray results, etc.) as well as on the experience of the clinician in applying similar therapies in like cases. Thus, the judgment that a given therapy is medically futile is a description of the objective quality of the therapy relative to a given patient in light of the patient's medical condition.[3] For this reason the determination that a therapy or medical intervention is medically futile rests with the physician alone. Once such a conclusion has been reached the physician should not be compelled either to offer or to provide the intervention.

This conclusion is challenged by those who argue that physicians and patients may value quite different outcomes in the medical encounter. While the physician may conclude that continued efforts to preserve the physiologic function of a person in irreversible coma are not justified, some patients and families may believe otherwise. Thus, in the case of Mrs. Wanglie, the family insisted that continued physiologic function was what they wanted even if maintained function could not serve Mrs. Wanglie's overall well-being. But the fact that a patient or family wants an outcome does not legitimate the pursuit of that outcome, particularly when such pursuit requires ongoing medical care provided by and within a community of person and the use of medical resources.

CONCLUSION

The determination that an available therapy is medically futile is a professional judgment based on verifiable medical data about the potential of a given intervention to affect the overall, integral well-being of the patient. This concern for and commitment to the good of the patient is at the heart of the medical profession. While individual physicians may have subjective feelings about particular patient outcomes (e.g., that life in persistent vegetative state is "not worth living") there is no evidence to suggest that determinations of medical futility, as in the Wanglie case, are shaped by the personal values of physicians. Neither should we conclude that reliance on physician judgment in determining medical futility threatens to undermine the rights and values of the patient or family in the care-giving relationship. Rather, supporting the physician in doing what she is educated to do in the context of the care-giving relationship ensures that patient good and well-being will continue to be at the heart of medical practice. The physician's role is to make reasoned decisions based on sound medical knowledge, to seek consultation to verify findings, and to recommend only those interventions that offer some reasonable hope of benefit. Compelling physicians to offer and provide therapies that, in their best medical judgment, are not conducive to the overall good of the patient risks changing the nature and focus of the care-giving relationship as well as the nature of the medical profession itself.

NOTES

1. R. Cranford, M.D., "Helga Wanglie's Ventilator." *Hastings Center Report* 21 (4): 23.

2. Academy of Neurology, "Statement on Certain Aspects of the Care and Management of the Persistent Vegetative State Patient." *Neurology* 1989 (39): 125–26.

3. Laurence Schneiderman, M.D., et al, "Medical Futility: Its Meaning and Ethical Implications," *Annals of Internal Medicine* 112 (12): 951.

36: Assessing Treatment Options: Recognizing the Limits

Over the past several years, there has been a growing disaffection for paternalism in medical practice among both physicians and patients. Underlying this disaffection has been an expanding societal awareness of and emphasis on individual rights and personal autonomy as well as the emergence of a better educated health care public. The result of these developments has been a recognition that decision making in health care is and must be a shared process between care provider and care receiver. Thus, patients and families are assuming a more active role in treatment decisions today than in the past. Within this changing environment some physicians are becoming unsure of the requirements of their role with regard to such decisions.[1]

Paralleling this development has been the rapid expansion of health care technologies. The scope of interventions available today includes: the ability to visualize and measure physiologic function in great detail; the capacity to gather, collate, and organize data to facilitate more efficient and comprehensive patient care; the ability to substitute for lost function and to circumvent the devastating effects of disease and disability. One predictable outcome of this development has been a growing reliance on the ability of available technologies to overcome the otherwise natural restrictions that are part of the human condition. However, the danger of allowing the technological imperative, i.e., the belief that if we can do something we must, to prescribe use of these technologies, looms large in health care today.

When these tracks converge, two potentially troubling situations can arise. On the one hand, the physician can approach the patient, or in the event of the patient's incapacity, the family or other appropriate surrogate, and offer a variety of available therapies from which to choose. "This is what we can do. What do you want us to do for you or your loved one?" In such an instance, patients and/or families are placed in the untenable position of having to make treatment decisions, a role for which they are neither prepared nor qualified. On the other hand, some physicians, fearful of the consequences of not giving adequate recognition to patient autonomy and self-determination, can find themselves ordering therapies that may not be medically indicated or appropriate but are provided because patients and/or families declare: "We want everything done!"

Neither approach is appropriate for neither recognizes the ethical limits associated with the goal of all decision making in health care, i.e., to contribute to the well-being of persons.

When a physician proposes some form of treatment to a patient, it should be with the hope that the regimen will provide benefit, i.e., that the patient will gain or at least maintain some ability to participate in and appreciate life and its attendant goods. In offering available treatment(s) to patients and/or families then, the physician ought to give the best possible projections about hoped for beneficial effects based on the physician's own considered judgment. That forecast certainly should include insight into the possible risks and/or burdens associated with the use of the therapy in question. Patients and families then weigh that information in light of their own values and goals and accept or refuse the proposed therapies.

But ought all available therapies be offered to patients and families? For example, should a patient who is in the terminal stages of cancer be offered CPR as a possibility in the event that cardiac/respiratory arrest occurs? Should renal dialysis be contemplated for the patient who has sustained profound and irreversible brain damage secondary to prolonged arrest? Should second or third liver transplants be made available to patients (or families) who have rejected the first liver and who are statistically less apt to benefit from repeated transplant attempts?

Often, lifesaving/sustaining therapies such as these are offered as possibilities to patients and families because the physician has failed to accept the responsibility to make some prior judgments about which of the available treatments are true options in a given case and which are not.

PRINCIPLES

In making determinations about which of the available therapies or treatments are real options, physicians should be guided by two basic ethical principles. First, beneficence should lead the physician to consider as viable choices only those therapies that offer some reasonable hope of providing benefit for the patient. Second, considerations of justice should prompt the care provider to recognize that in offering or providing therapies that are clearly non-beneficial, e.g., dialysis for a person in persistent vegetative state, not only can the patient be harmed rather than helped, but in addition, the broader society can be harmed because valuable and scarce resources can be wasted in the process.

Thus, some recognition of the limits that necessarily attend the practice of medicine, which ought to accompany the development and application of any medical technology, and which are a constitutive part of the human condition, must inform assessment of treatment options. In entering into the care-giving relationship with patients and families, care providers should spend some time discussing the boundaries of what is possible as well as what is beyond the realm of possibility in terms of treatment. Admittedly, these are difficult determinations to make. And it is equally difficult to discuss the necessary limitations with patients/families, many of whom have come to believe that nothing is impossible in health care today. However, to neglect (or worse to deny) that such limits do exist is to fail in the most basic obligation, i.e., always to care.

When cure or meaningful amelioration of the effects of disease or disability are no longer reasonably possible, the physician or other care provider is obliged to recognize that the limits have been met. Therapies that provide little or no hope of benefit ought not to be offered. Rather, the physician should exercise the responsibility that is hers and prepare the patient/family for approaching death in these circumstances. Admitting and accepting the limitations of available therapies precludes the inappropriate physician response: "Here is what we can do . . . you choose what you want us to do for you or your loved one." In addition, when patients and families demand "we want everything done," it allows for the more fitting response: "We have done everything possible. There is nothing more we can do."

CONCLUSION

Two principles, beneficence and justice, ought to be operative when the physician makes a determination about which treatments are truly viable options for a particular patient. The former focuses appropriately on patient need as the primary concern. The latter directs attention to the needs of the broader community and requires that, in treating individual patients, the community's resources be used appropriately. Thus, when an available treatment or therapy can offer no reasonable hope of benefiting the patient, it should not be offered as a possibility. If physicians fail to exercise appropriate responsibility in this regard, society will make such determinations for them. And when society makes these determinations, beneficence will not be the operative principle. Rather, economics will dictate treatment decisions.

NOTE

1. John Paris, SJ, Ph.D.; Robert Crone, M.D.; Frank Reardon, J.D., "Physicians' Refusal of Requested Treatment." *New England Journal of Medicine* 322 (14):1012–15.

37: Nancy Beth Cruzan Revisited*

Injured in an automobile accident in January, 1983, Nancy Beth Cruzan now lies in a persistent vegetative state and medical diagnosis concludes she will never recover her cognitive-affective function. The trial court of Jasper County, Judge Charles Teel, Jr. presiding, ruled on July 27, 1988 that the gastrostomy tube through which nutrition and hydration were being provided could be removed. However, on November 16, 1988, after agreeing that Nancy would never recover cognitive-affective function, the Supreme Court of Missouri determined in a 4–3 decision, that the ruling of the trial court should be reversed. Thus, the gastrostomy tube will remain in place, unless the decision is reversed by the United States Supreme Court.

PRINCIPLES

The decision of the Supreme Court of Missouri is subject to question on legal grounds.[1] For example, in contradiction to decisions in other states, the ruling denies that the constitutional right of privacy includes the right of a person to refuse medical treatment. Moreover, seemingly in contradiction to Living Will legislation approved by the State of Missouri, the Supreme Court declares that the state's interest in preserving life is unqualified, thus precluding "quality of life" factors from consideration when making decisions concerning withholding or withdrawing life support. However, in this essay we shall not consider the legal argumentation of the decision. The dissenting opinions offered by members of the Supreme Court have indicated the major difficulties in this regard. Rather, assuming that good legal decisions should be founded upon ethical reasoning as well as upon legal precedent, we shall consider the decision in the Cruzan case from an ethical perspective.

First of all, the Supreme Court decision continually describes the removal of the gastrostomy tube as causing the death of Nancy Beth Cruzan. If the family of Nancy Beth Cruzan was trying to cause her death, that indeed

---

*Editor's Note: This essay was written after November of 1988, when the Supreme Court of Missouri ruled that Nancy Beth Cruzan's life support could not be legally removed even though the medical diagnosis was that she could never recover cognitive-affective function. The salient ethical issues in the health care due to her and to others living in a similar, persistent vegetative state are herein carefully reviewed since the ethical reasoning of the Missouri Supreme Court is not acceptable.

would be ethically unacceptable. But their entire series of actions belie this interpretation. A more accurate description of the actions proposed by the Cruzan family would state that they wish to withdraw the gastrostomy tube because it is ineffective therapy and imposes a grave burden upon her. If the gastrostomy tube is removed, her death may be anticipated, but the *cause* of her death will be the underlying pathology (inability to swallow) that the gastrostomy tube has temporarily circumvented. This distinction between intending to kill (euthanasia) and withholding or withdrawing the means to prolong life when the means are ineffective or present a grave burden to the patient (an act of mercy) is accepted as standard in the ethics of health care.[2] The question the Court should ask, therefore, is: Are the means utilized to prolong Nancy's life ineffective or a grave burden for her? Language that indicates that the family is trying to bring about the death of their daughter is insensitive as well as misleading.

Though the Court does not ask the question explicitly, it implies that the means utilized to prolong Nancy's life are effective because it continually states: "She is not in a terminal condition and could live a long time". But this statement begs the question. All realize that with the gastrostomy tube in place, Nancy could live for a long time and, in this sense, is not in a terminal condition. But the question at issue is not how long Nancy will live with the tube in place. Rather, the question at issue is whether the gastrostomy tube should be removed, either because it is ineffective or imposes a grave burden upon Nancy Beth. The fact that the tube is already in place does not change the answer because there is no ethical difference between withholding and withdrawing life support.

DISCUSSION

In order to determine whether the gastrostomy tube is effective or ineffective, we must ask why it was implanted. Certainly it was not implanted to keep Nancy Beth in a persistent vegetative state. Rather, it was implanted when her condition was not clear and it was hoped that if nutrition and hydration were supplied, that some degree of cognitive-affective function would be restored. The present condition of Nancy Beth makes it clear that the tube in question is ineffective.

Does the continued use of the tube impose a grave burden upon Nancy Beth? When discussing this issue, the Court states that the gastrostomy tube is not "heroically invasive" nor "oppressively burdensome". But it is clear that the Court considers physical pain to be the only source of burden. The fact that the Cruzan family is burdened by the condition of Nancy is admitted by the Court, but is considered accidental to the issue under discussion. But in an ethical evaluation of burden to a patient, the consideration has never been limited to physical pain. Psychic pain is also to be considered as well as the burden to a family. Is not existing in a persistent vegetative state a psychic burden for a person? The whole purpose of making decisions for people who are incapable of making decisions is to make sure they are treated humanely as worthwhile human beings. People find psychic pain just as much a burden as physical pain. People across the country attest that they would want care withdrawn if it only prolongs existence in a totally debilitated state. Moreover, loving people consider their families when they make decisions about the burden of medical treatment. Proxies should do the same.

Another ethical issue not properly understood by the Court concerns proxy consent and justification for its use. As indicated above, proxy consent originates with the desire and responsibility to help people who cannot make decisions for themselves. Proxy consent is often offered for incompetent elderly people, but we realize the meaning and extent of this method of ensuring beneficial treatment for incapacitated people if we recall that the role of parents requires frequent exercise of proxy consent. Parents are assumed to act in a beneficent manner for their children. Only when their actions are patently or potentially harmful may agencies of the state intercede. The use of proxy consent flows from the very nature of human relationships, from a desire to ensure that the incompetent are treated with care and compassion. Given this natural right of loved ones to act on behalf of incompetent family members, it is startling to read in the Cruzan decision, "the guardian's power to exercise third party choice arises from the state's authority, not the constitutional right of the ward. The guardian is the delegate the state's *patrens patriae* power". The assumption that one needs the permission of the state in order to make decisions for an incompetent loved one is simply preposterous.

NOTES

1. Supreme Court of Missouri; "Cruzan vs. Harmon." Nov. 16, 1988.
2. President's Commission for the Study of Ethical Problems in Medicine and Behavioral Research. *Deciding to Forgo Life-Sustaining Treatment* (1983), 85.

38: Unfinished Business in the Cruzan Case*

In November of 1990, Charles Teel, judge of the circuit court of Jasper County in the state of Missouri, heard once again the petition of Joe and Joyce Cruzan to remove life support from their daughter Nancy Beth, who was seriously injured in an automobile accident in 1983. Declaring that there was "clear and convincing" evidence of her wishes not to exist in a persistent vegetative state, on December 14, Judge Teel declared that artificial hydration and nutrition could be withdrawn from Nancy Beth. Nancy Beth died of natural causes on December 26, 1990.

Unlike his response to a similar decision of Judge Teel in 1988, William Webster, the attorney general of Missouri, did not appeal the decision of 1990. He maintained that "The state is no longer interested in the Cruzan case." But allowing Nancy Beth Cruzan to die of natural causes was not the final curtain for the Cruzan case. There is some unfinished business. Namely, revoking the ethical reasoning the Supreme Court of Missouri expressed when reversing the original decision of Judge Teel. If the statements expressed by the Missouri Supreme Court in the original case are not explicitly renounced, many other families will experience the same anguish and suffering as did the Cruzans, and future legislation of Missouri in regard to removing life support will be flawed.

Clearly, decisions of courts are based more upon legal precedent than upon ethical reasoning. But some reliance upon ethical reasoning is required in order to formulate equitable court decisions. As the Missouri Supreme Court stated in the Cruzan case: "We remain true to our role only if our decision is firmly founded on legal principle *and reasoned analysis.*" Reasoned analysis is another term for ethical reasoning. What was the ethical reasoning underlying the Missouri Supreme Court decision in the Cruzan case?

*Editor's Note: This essay was written after the Supreme Court of Missouri's reversal in November of 1990 of its earlier 1988 ruling that denied removal of Nancy Beth Cruzan's life support. As in Essay 37, a careful review of the salient ethical issues in the health care due to her and others in similar vegetative state are seen in the light of the flawed ethical judgment still expressed by the reversal.

THREE ASSUMPTIONS

Three assumptions underlie the efforts of the court at ethical reasoning. All three assumptions seem deficient when examined in the light of ethical norms for removing life support from people who suffer from a fatal pathology. First of all, the court assumes that allowing a person to die because therapy is ineffective is the same as killing the person. The court stated: "This is not a case in which we are asked to let someone die. . . . This is a case in which we are asked to allow the medical profession to make Nancy die by starvation and dehydration." "Making someone die," or "causing the death" of another person means that the agent of the action intends the death of the other person and, by placing or omitting actions, brings about death. When a person will not benefit from medical care however, the intention of people removing the care is not to bring about death, but rather to admit that the illness or pathology threatening death cannot be treated in a manner that is beneficial for the patient. When life support is removed from a patient because it is not beneficial, we are simply admitting the limits of human ingenuity and medical science. How many times do people express their intentions when support is removed from loved ones, uttering such phrases as: "We cannot help Mom anymore;" or "Dad wouldn't want to live in this condition."

While the distinction between intending death and admitting human limitations is a fine one, it is realistic. Good ethical distinctions are thin as silk and strong as steel. In the case of persons in persistent vegetative state or in other conditions in which therapy is either ineffective or would impose a grave burden, removing life support does not *cause* death. Rather, removing life support allows death to occur as the result of a natural pathology that is not beneficial to resist. There is no moral imperative to prevent people from dying if they are in p.v.s. or suffer from other severely debilitating conditions from which they will not recover. Moreover, the court's statement that Nancy Beth would die of starvation and dehydration if life support were removed is inaccurate as well as inflammatory. This language brings to mind a vision of a conscious and healthy person dying an excruciating death because she is deprived of beneficial care. Reference to "starvation and dehydration" of p.v.s. patients has little relation to reality. People in p.v.s. die because of injury to their cerebral cortex. Just as they can no longer chew or swallow, so they do not feel pain.[1]

The second assumption underlying the decision of the Missouri Supreme Court in the Cruzan case is that persons suffering from fatal pathologies must be kept alive as long as possible. The Court expresses this assumption by consistently referring to the fact that Nancy "is not terminally ill" and for this reason would not allow removal of life support. Others repeated this error by stating: "Nancy is not dying." But both statements imply that Nancy's fatal pathology would be assessed ethically only *after* life support has been utilized. To be "terminally ill" in the mind of the Missouri Supreme Court means that a person will die *even if* life support has been applied. According to this assumption respirators, dialysis, and especially artificial hydration and nutrition should not be removed unless they fail to prolong life. But when assessing whether or not to use or continue life support, the essential question is not *if* life can be prolonged, but rather *should* life be prolonged. Will the person benefit if life is prolonged? In ethical reasoning the questions "will the life support impose a grave burden, and will the life support be effective" are asked before life support is utilized. The Illinois Supreme Court recently presented a more accurate interpretation of terminal illness. It stated: "If the very delay caused by the procedures were allowed to govern the assessment of imminence, the definition of a terminal illness would be rendered circular and meaningless and make it impossible for compassionate care for people unable to benefit from therapy. *Imminence must be judged as if the death delaying procedures were absent*".[2] Hopefully, this insight in regard to "terminal illness," which is more in accord with ethical reasoning will become accepted across the country. If so, much of the misunderstanding and contention that surrounds the removal of life support should be obviated.

The third assumption underlying the Court's decision was that "The state's interest is not in the quality of life. The state's interest is an unqualified interest in life." If quality of life implies impaired function due to serious pathology, and if the state has no interest in quality of life, then every means possible must be utilized in order to prolong the life of every person suffering from any impaired function whatsoever. How severely impaired the person might be would not matter, as long as the person could be kept alive. According to this thinking, we should consider kidney transplants for people in p.v.s. who have end stage renal disease and heart transplants for people in p.v.s. who have chronic cardiomyopathy. These conclusions are ludicrous but in accord with the Court's reasoning. All other state courts that have rendered decisions in p.v.s. cases have admitted a reasonable limit to state interest in the face of seriously impaired function. As Judge Blackmar pointed out in his dissent to the majority opinion in the Cruzan case, if Missouri has an unqualified interest in preserving life, how to explain the existence of capital punishment and the Living Will law in Missouri.

CONCLUSION

The "reasoned analysis" of the Missouri Supreme Court in the Cruzan case should be analyzed and improved in the light of basic ethical principles. Until it is, there is unfinished business in the Cruzan case. But in a certain sense, the decisions of the court and the supporting argumentation are beside the point. More important is the question: Is the court the place to decide questions which concern prolonging life for persons severely debilitated as the result of fatal pathologies? Questions of this nature have been settled in the family forum for years. Does the court do a better job than the family? The family forum is public; not only family members but physicians, nurses, clergy, and others are involved in the ultimate decision. Moreover, the family forum has a more humane and compassionate motivation than the legal forum. Rather than being mainly concerned with state interest and legal precedent, the family forum is concerned with doing what is best for the patient.

NOTES

1. "Position of the American Academy of Neurology on certain aspects of the care and management of the persistent vegetative state patient." *Neurology* 39, January 1989, 125–27.
2. Supreme Court of Illinois, "In re Estate of Sidney Greenspan"; July 9, 1990, 15.

39: Care for Patients in Persistent Vegetative State

The diagnosis, prognosis, and care of patients who are in a persistent vegetative state (p.v.s.), has been the issue underlying much ethical and legal controversy. The decision of the Massachusetts Supreme Court in the Brophy case, and the decision of the Missouri Supreme Court in the Cruzan case, were diametrically opposed. Yet both Courts sought to base their decisions on the medical care suitable for patients in p.v.s. Ethicists are also divided in regard to the proper care for patients in p.v.s. Some ethicists maintain that all patients who are in p.v.s. should receive artificial hydration and nutrition because they will benefit from such treatment. Others maintain that such treatment is optional for patients in this condition because, even though artificial hydration and nutrition circumvents a fatal pathology and extends life, it does not offer an overall benefit to the patient. In this essay, we shall present briefly the statement of the American Academy of Neurology in regard to people in p.v.s. (*Neurology*, January, 1989, 39) and offer some ethical observations.

PRINCIPLES

The statement may be divided into three main sections: the medical description of a person in p.v.s.; the nature of artificial hydration and nutrition; and the use of artificial nutrition and hydration for a person in p.v.s.

1. *The medical description.* The patient who is in p.v.s. is permanently unconscious as a result of a functioning brain stem and a total loss of cerebral cortical functioning. Usually the person is able to breathe spontaneously, but has no self-awareness; he is unable to perform voluntary actions and does not experience pain. The diagnosis of such a condition can be made with a high degree of medical certainty after a period of one to three months. Patients in a persistent vegetative state may continue to survive for a prolonged period of time as long as artificial provision of nutrition and fluids is continued. Thus, because life support has been utilized, patients in this condition are not "terminally ill." But the condition described above is permanent because of the trauma and total loss of function in the cerebral cortex.

2. *The nature of artificial hydration and nutrition.* The artificial provision of hydration and nutrition is a medical treatment rather than a nursing

procedure, and is analogous to other forms of life-sustaining treatment, such as a respirator. When a patient is unconscious, both a respirator and an artificial feeding device serve to support or replace normal bodily functions that are compromised as a result of the patient's illness.

3. *The use of artificial hydration and nutrition for patients in p.v.s.* It is good medical practice to initiate hydration and nutrition when the patient's prognosis is uncertain, but to allow for termination if the patient's condition is hopeless, the family having been informed and consented to the withdrawal. Artificial hydration and nutrition may be discontinued in accordance with the principles and practices governing the withholding and withdrawing of the forms of medical treatment, i.e., based on a careful evaluation of the patient's diagnosis and prognosis, the prospective benefits and burdens of the treatment, and the stated preferences of the patient and family. When medical treatment fails to promote a patient's well-being, there is no longer any ethical obligation to provide it. Medical treatment, including the medical provision of artificial nutrition and hydration, provides no hope for benefit to patients in p.v.s. once the diagnosis has been established to a high degree of medical certainty.

DISCUSSION

Several points in this statement are relevant from an ethical perspective.

1. This is an ethical statement by physicians concerning an important and difficult issue in medical care. For this reason alone, it is worthy of note. For too long judges, lawyers, theologians, and ethicists have analyzed contentious issues in medicine and many scientists and physicians have acted as though their profession were "value free." While not denying the contribution of ethics and law to the solution of issues arising from medical care, the voice of medicine must be heard also if a well-balanced and clinical view of these human problems is to develop. Hopefully, physicians' groups will apply themselves to other ethical issues associated with medicine, such as the access to health care.

2. The statement and proof that artificial hydration and nutrition is a medical treatment similar to the use of a respirator is welcome because it offers a model for decision making that most people can understand. The great contribution of the A.A.N. statement, though, is the simple syllogism: Medical treatment attempts to promote the well-being of the patient. But artificial hydration and nutrition does not promote the well-being of a person in p.v.s. Therefore, artificial hydration and

nutrition may be withheld from a patient who is in a persistent vegetative state.

3. There is no hint of approval of euthanasia, neither active nor passive, in this statement. The reason for withdrawing treatment from a patient permanently unconscious is not a quality of life argument. Rather, treatment is withdrawn by analyzing the quality of the means insofar as the condition of the patient is concerned. When artificial hydration and nutrition are withdrawn, the family and physicians do not intend death and do not *cause* death. Rather, death is *caused* by the underlying pathology; the inability to chew and swallow. The intention of the family and physician is to avoid doing something that would be useless or that would impose an excessive burden on the patient.

4. Grasping the distinction between avoiding harm to the patient (a good act) and *causing* the patient's death (an evil act) is difficult for many when artificial hydration and nutrition are in question. The main reason for this difficulty seems to be that death occurs inevitably when the artificial hydration and nutrition are removed, no matter what the motive underlying the removal might be. But human actions receive their designation as good or evil from the effect of the action and the intention of the person performing or withholding the action, not from the accidental effects of the action. Hence, if the proximate motive of removing the hydration and nutrition is to avoid harming the patient, then the ensuing death, because it is not intended, is extraneous to the moral evaluation of the act. One way to help people make a good ethical decision about removing life support is to ask: "Would you remove this life support even if it would not result in the patient's death?"

CONCLUSION

For many reasons, the statement of the A.A.N. is welcome and enlightening. But the statement alone will not lead to consensus. Rather, we need more discussion and common understanding of such terms as the quality of life, the nature of a moral act, what constitutes the well-being of a patient and causing death as distinguished from allowing death to occur naturally when there is no moral imperative to prolong life.

40: Use of Artificial Hydration and Nutrition: The Clouds Are Lifting

For the past ten years, the use of artificial hydration and nutrition (a.h.n.) for patients in a persistent vegetative state (p.v.s.) has been the subject of ethical and legal dispute. In the Catholic tradition, for example, some maintained that removing a.h.n. from any patient was unethical because it was the same as starving a person to death. For them, withdrawal of artificial hydration and nutrition would always be murder or euthanasia. Others maintained that while it was possible in theory to withdraw a.h.n. from p.v.s. patients, in practice it should not be allowed because use of a.h.n. did not constitute a grave burden for the p.v.s. patient and should be considered effective therapy because it sustained life, albeit at a low level of function. Still others maintained that the traditional teaching of the Church allowed the removal of a.h.n. from patients in p.v.s. They maintained that p.v.s. involves a lethal pathology (inability to chew and swallow) and that circumvention of the pathology through a.h.n. imposes a grave burden (at least upon the family and perhaps society), or that such therapy is ineffective insofar as the purpose of life is concerned.

In the realm of legal reasoning, courts in various states handled the situation differently. Courts in New Jersey and Massachusetts for example, allowed the withdrawal of a.h.n. from patients in p.v.s. at the request of family members, reasoning that the family members were capable of expressing the wishes of incapacitated persons. In Missouri, and to a certain extent in New York, the state courts rejected the family testimony as evidence sufficient to prove the wishes of incapacitated persons. The Supreme Court of Missouri stated that "clear and convincing evidence" of the p.v.s. patient's desire must be presented before a.h.n. could be removed. While the Missouri Supreme Court did not define clear and convincing evidence, it was clear that the incapacitated person's previous statements to family members did not suffice.

While the dispute concerning the use of artificial hydration and nutrition is far from over, as a result of some recent statements by the magisterium of the Church, and the recent decision of the United States Supreme Court, the solution to the question is becoming more clear.

PRINCIPLES

Recent statements by Bishop John Leibrecht[1] of Springfield, MO, the local bishop of the region in Missouri where the Cruzans live, and by the bishops of the Texas Catholic Conference[2] have clarified the issue for Catholic teaching. While not adding anything new to the dialogue, these statements confirm that removal of a.h.n. from p.v.s. patients is in accord with the traditional Catholic teaching. In the course of their statement, the Texas Bishops, agreeing with several medical societies, acknowledge that p.v.s. patients "are stricken with a lethal pathology." From the ethical perspective, this is a fundamental fact. This fact differentiates the withholding of food and water from people in p.v.s. from withholding food and water from infants, retarded adults, and other disabled people who do not have a lethal pathology but need assistance in obtaining nutrition and hydration. Clearly, the lethal pathology of the p.v.s. patient may be circumvented by means of a.h.n. But is there a moral obligation to circumvent the lethal pathology? Only if it is truly beneficial for the total well-being of the patient.

    While the decision of the United States Supreme Court in the Cruzan case did not provide immediate relief for Nancy Beth Cruzan or the Cruzan family, it did dispose for more rational procedures in the future. First of all, the court declared that from a legal perspective, a.h.n. is a medical therapy, thus implying that it should be subject to the burden/benefit analysis utilized when judging any medical therapy. Second, in allowing the withdrawal of life support from an incapacitated person, the court recognized the difference between killing a person and allowing the person to die when therapy is no longer beneficial. Third, even though the court allowed Missouri to require "clear and convincing evidence" that a person in a p.v.s. would want life support removed, the court implied that other states could require a less stringent standard of evidence, such as living wills or durable powers of attorney. Indeed, an individual state could even decide to allow decisions concerning use or withdrawal of life support to be made in the family forum by loved ones and medical care givers. This method of decision making was accepted in the United States before the Karen Quinlan case and is followed today throughout most of the world.

    In not extending to the other states the stringent requirements for evidence developed by the Missouri Supreme Court, the United States Supreme Court eviscerated the decision of the Missouri Supreme Court. Recall that the legal decision of the Missouri Supreme Court was based upon ethical reasoning that did not recognize the important distinctions that must be utilized in cases of this kind; e.g., (1) "But this is not a case in which we are asked to allow someone to die . . . Nancy is not terminally ill . . . this is a case in which we are asked to allow the medical profession to make Nancy die by starvation and dehydration." (2) "Life is precious and worthy of preservation without regard to its quality." (3) "A guardian's power to exercise third-party choice arises from the state's authority, not the Constitutional right of the ward." Indeed, the ethical reasoning of the Missouri Supreme Court seemed to indicate that a.h.n. should never be removed from p.v.s. patients. Clearly, the United States Supreme Court does not agree that removing a.h.n. from Nancy Beth Cruzan is killing her, did not affirm that the quality of life is a meaningless consideration when determining the removal of life support, and did not absolutize the rights of a state-appointed guardian. Given the situation in Missouri, it seems a propitious time for the legislature to enact some reasonable norms in regard to removing life support from p.v.s. patients.

DISCUSSION

Can any practical norms be developed as a result of these recent documents? It seems the following conclusions may be drawn:

1. When making moral or ethical decisions concerning the removal of a.h.n. from p.v.s. patients, one may not say that such an action is contrary to Catholic teaching. If a.h.n. imposes a grave burden upon a p.v.s. patient, or is judged ineffective therapy for the integral well-being of the patient, then it may be withdrawn.
2. The evidence that will demonstrate that a p.v.s. patient would want a.h.n. withdrawn were he or she able to express an opinion will vary from one state to another. Some states will recommend the use of living wills or durable power of attorney in order to establish evidence. Other states will accept the testimony of family if it is coupled with court approved medical testimony that a lethal pathology exists. Still other states, imitating the custom in most of the civilized world, will allow loved ones and care givers to make decisions for incapacitated persons.
3. When faced with decisions concerning removal of a.h.n. or any life support, care givers and administrators of health care facilities should be concerned with the total well-being of the patient and the patient's family, rather than with avoiding litigation. While the two goods are not incompatible, many care givers and administrations of health care facilities often follow the advice of house counsel and gear all their actions to avoiding litigation. Time after time, physicians and CEOs of health care facilities have refused to remove life-support systems unless there is a court order to do so. My point is not to ignore the

law, but to insist that compassionate patient care can be achieved while avoiding litigation.

NOTES

1. Bishop John Leibrecht "The Nancy Cruzan Case," *Origins* 1/11/90, 525–26.
2. Pastoral Statement on Artificial Hydration and Nutrition, *Origins*, 6/7/90, p. 53ff.

41: Living Will and Durable Power of Attorney

In the last ten years, several prominent court cases have been concerned with the removal of life support from people no longer able to make medical decisions for themselves. As people discuss the Quinlan, Brophy, O'Connor, Cruzan, and Busalacchi cases, they affirm the desire to avoid such disputes if they would ever be in the same condition as the aforementioned people. In order to facilitate the desire to avoid unwanted therapy, many states have approved the use of living wills (LW) and durable powers of attorney (DPA) for health affairs. Both documents allow persons while still competent to express the way in which they would like medical care to be rendered when they are incapacitated, that is, no longer capable of medical decision making. Usually, the decision that a person is incapacitated is made by one or two physicians. These documents exonerate the persons who implement them from any civil or criminal liability. In general, the LW is implemented by an attending physician, and the DPA is implemented by a proxy, known as the agent or attorney-in-fact. The LW is to be implemented when death threatens and the person is incapable of medical decision making. The DPA is implemented as soon as the person becomes incapable of medical decision making; it is operative if death does not threaten or if it does threaten. While both documents are inherently ethical, they are often ineffective in accomplishing the goals that people have in mind when they sign them. In this essay, we shall seek to explain the difficulties involved in the use of both documents and offer some suggestions that may alleviate the difficulties.

DIFFICULTIES

Some believe that life support may not be withheld or removed if a patient has not signed a LW or DPA. But even if the LW or DPA were not signed by the patient, the ethical right to withhold or remove life support that is no longer beneficial must be recognized. In other words, though a clearly written LW or DPA may facilitate the removal of life support, the moral right of a family, in collaboration with the attending physician, to determine when life support is a grave burden or is useless is still an ethical means of decision making for an incapacitated person. We receive the ethical responsibility to make decisions concerning our own health care and the health care of our incapacitated loved ones from our nature as human beings. The Constitution

141

and state laws may recognize and structure our decision making rights, but they do not create these rights. Hence, the LW and DPA may facilitate good decision making, but they do not create the moral power to make such decisions.

Though most state laws concerning LW and DPA allow persons to write their own documents, these state laws usually contain model forms for people to sign while still competent. The wording of these model forms often gives rise to ambiguity and ethical questions. For example: Most LW legislation states that the document is to be implemented when the patient is in "a terminal condition," and allows the removal of life support when it "only prolongs the process of dying." But what is the meaning of "terminal condition?" Many state laws define terminal condition as an illness from which death will result in a relatively short time, *even if life support has been utilized.* According to this interpretation, life support can be removed only if death is deemed imminent. Death is not deemed imminent if life support will sustain even a minimal degree of function. A more realistic definition of terminal illness has recently been offered by the Illinois Supreme Court (Greenspan Case). To date, however, it is not widely accepted. Moreover, the phrase "only prolongs the process of dying" is medically meaningless. When applying life support, reputable physicians seek to restore human function; not to "prolong the process of dying."

As a result of the ambiguous language cited above, the LW was ineffective and has been supplanted in many states by the DPA for health affairs. By reason of the DPA, the agent usually is given the power to make all health care decisions for the now incapacitated person, even if the patient is not in a terminal condition. In some states confinement to a mental institution or an electroconvulsive therapy requires a court order in addition to a decision by the agent.

The greatest potential difficulty of the DPA is found in the section that indicates that the agent will make health care decisions in accord with the values and principles that the patient would follow were he or she capable of decision making. This presupposes that the person making the DPA has thought through his or her desires and communicated them to the agent. But just as a marriage license does not ensure the existence of marital love, so a DPA document does not ensure that the proper communication has taken place.

Clearly, the agent is given extensive powers of decision making through the DPA. But what about the responsibilities of the physician? Physicians are also patient advocates, not blind servants of surrogate decision makers. Ethical health care for incapacitated patients with a DPA will still require cooperation between physicians and surrogates. While some physicians have welcomed the DPA because it frees them from legal liability and enables them to work with a definite person as surrogate, it does not free them from ethical responsibilities. Physicians must still offer and implement plans for medical treatment in accord with the overall well-being of the patient.

SUGGESTIONS

There are no easy solutions to the above mentioned difficulties, but the following suggestions may be of some help.

1. Keep in mind that medical decisions may be made for incapacitated patients even if they have not filled out a LW or DPA. These decisions, made in collaboration with the attending physician, should be made by loved ones, using the ethical norms followed for centuries. "If able to make a decision, what would mom or dad want in these circumstances?"

2. Because the interpretation of the LW is sometimes ambiguous, utilize the DPA, making it fulfill the goals of the LW. Hence, state explicitly that the DPA will be effective at all times, even as death approaches.

3. Be sure to discuss your desires and values with the person you designate as agent. In this discussion, focus on the mental and physical functions you consider necessary for a meaningful life; that is, point out the impairments and disabilities that would justify withholding or removing life support; e.g., if you have advanced Alzheimer's disease, do you wish to be treated for pneumonia? If you have not thought through your values and desires, perhaps you would ask your proxy to act in accord with the teaching of your church in regard to the use and removal of life support.

4. Realize that you can state reservations in your DPA; e.g., will you allow your agent to commit you to a mental institution without a court order?

5. Avoid mentioning specific medical treatments that you wish excluded in the event you are incapacitated. The very therapy you exclude, (e.g. artificial hydration and nutrition) may be the therapy that will restore you to decision making capacity. Instead, encourage life support, but include the desire to have it removed if it does not restore function that would be essential for you to pursue the purpose of life.

CONCLUSION

The ethical norms for medical care and life prolonging therapy are clear; life should be prolonged unless the therapy to prolong life imposes a grave burden or is ineffective insofar as the overall well-being of the patient is concerned. Used wisely, the DPA follows these norms. Moreover, it can keep decision making out of the legal forum and in the family forum, where it belongs.

42: Coming Soon to Your Neighborhood Health Care Facility: The Patient Self-determination Act

The Patient Self Determination Act (PSDA), went into effect in December, 1991, and has changed considerably the manner in which health care facilities offer patient care. The overall purpose of the act is to increase the use of advance directives for health care. In the previous essay the merits of two most common forms of advanced directives, the Living Will and the Durable Power of Attorney, are discussed (p. 141–143). In this essay, we consider briefly the main provisions of the PSDA and more extensively some ethical issues to which the legislation may give rise.

PRINCIPLES

The main provisions of the PSDA affecting health care facilities and physicians are:

1. Every health care facility that receives Medicare or Medicaid funding from the federal government must give to each incoming patient a statement of rights in regard to making health care decisions. Thus, the bill applies to hospitals, nursing homes, home health agencies, hospice programs, and HMOs. The statement of rights will be derived from the law and court decisions of the state in which the facility is located.
2. The health care facility also must ask patients if they have advance directives. If a person has made an advance directive, this fact must be documented in the medical record. Possibly, the simplest way to fulfill this stipulation is to place a copy of the advance directive in the patient's chart. If the patient has not executed an advance directive, this fact also must be documented, but health care may not be withheld for that reason.
3. The facility must also give the patient an explanation of its own policy in regard to advance directives. If the provisions of the advance directives of the patient violate the policies of the facility, the patient

144

must be informed that some stipulations of the advance directives will not be honored. For example, if an advance directive calls for physician-assisted euthanasia, facilities that oppose such a practice should have a statement prepared in advance that explains that advance directives containing such requests will not be honored.

4. The health care facility must "ensure compliance with the requirements of state law." For this purpose, the facility has the duty to provide education programs for staff and community regarding advance directives and their meaning. Clearly physicians, as well as other health care professionals, will need instructions concerning effective implementation of advance directives.

DISCUSSION

At least three significant ethical issues may arise as the result of this legislation:

1. If they have not done so already, some patients may wish to execute advance directives at the time of admission to the health care facility. Because of the tension, anxiety, and depression experienced by many people when they are admitted to a nursing home, hospital, or hospice program, this is a poor time to make decisions concerning future health care. Moreover, advance directives should be made after prudent reflection and from a perspective of faith. To allow patients to prepare hurriedly advance directives fosters the depersonalization of medicine. In general then, it would be beneficial for all concerned if the advance directive were executed well before patients are admitted to health care facilities. If a patient has not executed an advance directive and requests to do so at the time of admission, it would seem more helpful to persuade the person to delay the process. If a patient were to insist on executing a directive at the time of admission, it seems the facility should provide counseling in regard to the meaning and effects of the document.

2. Because an advance directive is such an important document, the person who will make health care decisions for an incapacitated person should know the goals and wishes of the person who has executed the document. Often, the communication between the person who executes the advance directive and the person who will ensure compliance with it is weak or nonexistent. How can one act as a reputable agent for another unless the proxy is able to "stand in the shoes" of the patient? Studies show that decisions of proxies are inaccurate if effective communication has not taken place. If communication between patients and the persons who will become their agents is nonexis-

tent or weak, then the process of decision making may become a legalistic farce.

The need for communication between patient and proxy is also obvious if advance directives have *not* been executed. Legislation authorizing advance directives does not *create* the right of proxy decision making. Rather, such legislation merely *regulates* this right of proxy decision making and seeks to make the exercise of this right more effective. The proxy for a person who has not executed an advance directive usually will be a family member. Unless some serious conversation has taken place concerning the wishes of the patient, the proxy will be left without any objective evidence for decision making. The use of artificial nutrition and hydration for example, should be discussed explicitly. People with a living faith will do well to discuss the implications of their faith with family members so that decisions concerning the prolongation of life will be formulated in accord with their religious beliefs.

3. Potentially, the most serious ethical issue resulting from the PSDA is the implied assumption that physicians are simply to carry out the wishes of the proxy or attorney-in-fact. Physicians have a moral responsibility to listen to the requests of proxies, but they also have a moral responsibility to do what is "good" for the patient. The "good" of the patient is derived from an appreciation of the patient's value system *and* from the knowledge and skill of medicine. Thus, though a proxy or attorney-in-fact may convey accurately the patient's stated requests, these requests are to be interpreted in light of information only physicians are able to supply. A recent case illustrates this issue: When Sam, a young man in a coma as a result of an automobile accident, was brought to the emergency room, his family told the trauma surgeons that Sam had stated he never wanted a respirator or artificial hydration and nutrition to be used in his behalf. The physicians countered: "If we don't use these life supports Sam will die, and we have seen people in worse conditions eventually walk out of here." After some persuasion, the family consented to the use of both ventilator and artificial hydration and nutrition. The happy ending of the story is that Sam did recover and walked out of a "rehab" center four months later. However, the essential issue in this case is not the success of the therapy. Rather, it is the nature of the decision that must be made when caring for seriously debilitated persons. Certainly, an attorney-in-fact has the right to request removal of life support that is a grave burden or that is ineffective. But therapy cannot be judged to be a grave burden or ineffective unless the medical condition of the patient and the hope for recovery (diagnosis and prognosis) are

known. Supplying this information is the responsibility of the physician.

Anyone associated with health care knows that incapacitated patients are often maintained on life support when it is no longer beneficial for them. In these cases, the "good" of the patient is equated sometimes with prolonging life, no matter what the quality of function. But in spite of these obvious cases of "overcare," the nature of the decision to utilize or remove life support must be portrayed accurately. More often than not, physicians continue life support because there seems to be some hope of restoring the incapacitated patient to a quality of function that the patient would consider beneficial. Medicine is not an exact science and the patient must be given the benefit of the doubt. When the PSDA was being discussed prior to approval by the U.S. Senate, the statement was often heard: "Thirty percent of Medicare funds are expended upon people in the last month of their lives." While the statistics may be accurate, it should be realized that this is a retrospective judgment. If physicians knew which patients would die in spite of aggressive and expensive care, the decision to withhold or remove life support would be much less complicated. But because medicine is an art as well as a science, the outcome of aggressive therapy is not predictable. Hence, determining what is "good" for the patient requires more than the statement of a proxy or attorney-in-fact.

CONCLUSION

While an advance directive is a useful and beneficial method of exercising one's natural right to make decisions concerning health care, perhaps the sledgehammer approach of the PSDA will cause more problems than it solves. Clearly, medical care should be withheld and life support should be removed if they are not beneficial for the patient. However, deciding what is beneficial is an act of love on the part of the proxy and an act of advocacy on the part of the physician. Both love and advocacy are frustrated unless adequate communication and empathy precede medical decision making.

43: Ethics Consultants and the Care-giving Relationship

Throughout the history of medicine, the goal of the physician has been described in terms of "contributing to the well-being of the patient" or of "doing good" for the patient. In other words, the practice of medicine has been understood, at least implicitly, as an ethical endeavor. Ethics is pervasive. Thus, many physicians practice ethics without realizing it. Today, however, there is a growing tendency to isolate certain circumstances or events as they occur in the ongoing care of a patient and to refer to this isolated happenings as the "ethical issues" or "ethical dilemmas," giving the impression that the ethical is episodic rather than pervasive. This proclivity fosters a lack of appreciation for the inherently ethical nature of the physician-patient relationship. One result of this mistaken tendency is to exempt the physician from the responsibility of ongoing ethical analysis and discourse in the care-giving relationship and to encourage reliance on specialists, i.e., ethics consultants. The paradigm for this approach is the use of specialists as consultants in other areas of medicine.

Coupled with the constant growth of scientific knowledge and expanding technological capabilities, the complexities of the human being make a comprehensive grasp of all the available information needed to respond to the medical needs of every patient a difficult task. As a result, the appropriateness of and need for specialists within medicine is widely accepted today. When a specialist is engaged as a consultant in the care of a given patient, her role and responsibilities are related to and derived from her particular area of expertise and the fact that certain aspects of medical knowledge and skill are beyond the competency of the physician seeking the consultation. Thus, if a gynecologist encounters a patient who demonstrates symptoms suggestive of right-sided heart failure, he may request that a cardiologist review the case to confirm the suspected diagnosis. Further, he may ask the specialist to assume responsibility for the care of the patient with relation to the cardiovascular problem. The reasonableness of this kind of arrangement is attested to by the realization that the primary physician cannot be expected to master the intricacies of cardiology in addition to his own area of expertise and competency. However, when the primary physician requests the services of a specialist there is no expectation that the specialist will try to help the primary physician gain a better understanding of the specialty. In many cases, there is little communication between the primary physician and the consultant save

148

what occurs in the medical record of the patient. Neither is there any expectation that calling upon a specialist to help with the care of the patient will increase the primary physician's ability to handle similar cases in the future. The need for the specialist exists because the primary physician has chosen not only to focus on his particular area of interest in medicine, but also to exclude from his competency other areas of medical practice. This is not to say that, given the appropriate training, the primary physician lacks the ability to understand or practice cardiology or any other medical specialty. But because of the amount and complexity of medical knowledge, it is legitimate and indeed necessary for a physician to limit the scope of his endeavors to one area of medicine to the exclusion of many others.

Such an exclusionary option, however, must not be exercised with regard to the ethical in medicine. Ethics is not one specialty among many others in medicine. Rather, medicine is itself an ethical enterprise and the physician is obliged to consider and address the ethical in caring for every patient. Admittedly, many physicians are not conversant with the ethical principles that should inform the practice of medicine. Some physicians may be ill-equipped to discuss values and goods with patients and families in the process of discerning what will contribute to the patient's well-being. It should not be concluded, however, that the "ethical issues" that arise in the care of a patient can be turned over to an ethics specialist or consultant for scrutiny in the same manner as that described above in regard to medical specialist. The ethics consultant does have a role to play in helping physicians and other health care professionals address specific ethical concerns which arise in the care-giving relationship. But the appropriate role and responsibilities of the specialist in ethics is quite different from that of specialist in medicine. The difference must be appreciated if the integrity of medicine and the care-giving relationship are to be maintained.

DISCUSSION

When physician-initiated, most requests for ethics consultations occur because the physician is not clear about his ethical obligations in a given clinical situation. Thus, the primary role and function of the ethics consultant in medicine and health care is to "facilitate moral reflection and inquiry."[1] That is, the ethicist seeks to enable health care professionals to identify, reflect on, and deliberate their own ethical obligations as they arise in the care of patients. The ethicist helps physicians and others recognize the ethical principles and norms that guide decision making in medical practice in a way that makes it clear that these principles are derived from reflection on the meaning of medicine and the care-giving relationship. While there is a body of knowledge that justifies calling medical ethics a distinct discipline, the ethics consultant does not bring something new to the practice of medicine from outside, but rather, serves to focus on what is already an integral aspect of medical practice. Neither does the ethics consultant make decisions about specific ethical questions or issues that arise in the care of a patient. The ethicist's role is to elucidate the norms and principles that should guide decision making, clarify issues when necessary, and offer support to the physician and others who are involved in the decision-making process.

Finally, the ethics consultant should never encourage or foster dependence on her expertise in the area of ethics. Unlike the cardiologist who appropriately assumes responsibility for one aspect of the patient's care when requested to do so by the primary physician, the ethicist's role is to help care givers assume and exercise their own responsibility and judgment about the ethical issues in the care of the patient.

CONCLUSION

The nature of medicine and medical practice require that health care professionals appreciate and respond to the ethical dimension that provides the context for the care-giving relationship. The ethicist's role is to facilitate that appreciation and response by the physician and other specialist/consultant in order to educate care givers in the clinical setting so that they themselves can make decisions that contribute to the well-being of their patients.

NOTE

1. Terrence F. Ackerman, "Conceptualizing the Role of the Ethics Consultant: Some Theoretical Issues," in *Ethics Consultation in Health Care*, John Fletcher, ed. (Ann Arbor: Health Administration Press, 1989), 38.

44: Ethics Committees in Hospitals

Recently, the American Hospital Association (AHA) recommended that each hospital institute an ethics committee. Perhaps the action of the AHA is due to the study of ethics committees published by the President's Commission for Ethics in Medicine and Behavioral and Biomedical Research. Although the President's Commission stopped short of recommending that an ethics committee be established in each hospital, it clearly recommended that education, consultation, and review be available in each hospital for difficult decisions of patient care. The Joint Commission for the Accreditation of Health Care Facilities (JCAHF) also requires the availability of ethical consultation. Because of the recommendations of the three above-mentioned influential groups, this essay will be devoted to a consideration of the purpose and functions of ethics committees in hospitals and to evaluate their usefulness.

PRINCIPLES

Ethics committees in hospitals received their main impetus from the decision of the New Jersey Supreme Court in the Karen Quinlan case. The court, assuming erroneously that most hospitals had ethics committees, declared that such committees rather than the courts should be involved in decisions concerning withdrawal of life-support systems. In analyzing the hospital ethics committee, the President's Commission lists six potential functions:

1. Review a case to confirm the physician's diagnosis or prognosis of a patient's condition.
2. Review decisions made by physicians or surrogates about specific treatment.
3. Make decisions about suitable treatment for incompetent patients.
4. Provide general educational programs for staff on how to identify and solve ethical issues.
5. Formulate policies to be followed by staff in certain difficult cases.
6. Serve as consultant for physicians, patients, or their families in making specific ethical decisions.

DISCUSSION

Clearly, the last three functions are of an educational nature and they could be carried out in regard to routine ethical issues as well as in crisis situations. The first three functions are not educational; rather, they could be termed jurisdictional powers because they bespeak a review power and, in some cases, a decision-making power. These jurisdictional powers are needed, the commission maintains, in ethical cases that involve the medical treatment of incompetent patients who are in danger of death. For example, the ethics committee with these powers might be called on to affirm or deny the medical opinions that a patient is in a coma, to make a decision about withdrawing life-support equipment, or to review the decision-making process to ensure that all concerned people were consulted.

The Quinlan court and the AHA are interested in having hospitals form ethics committees with jurisdictional powers. The main concern of the court seems to be that cases concerning treatment for incompetent moribund patients be settled in the hospitals and not referred to the courts. One concern of the AHA seems to be that costs be controlled by removing life-support systems as soon as possible, while necessary safeguards to avoid malpractice suits are observed. Although the concerns of the court and the AHA are legitimate, there are definite difficulties that accompany giving jurisdictional power to a committee within a hospital. First, it may remove the medical and ethical decisions from the persons who are responsible for the decisions. In caring for dying people, whether competent or incompetent, physicians have the responsibility to make ethical decisions based on medical facts. The responsibility for discerning these medical facts cannot be given to other persons nor to a committee. The patient, or the patient's family if the patient is incompetent, also has ethical responsibilities that should not be delegated.

Second, giving review or decision-making power to the ethics committee may dilute the ethical decision-making process rather than improve it by weakening concern for the good of the patient. Everybody's business is nobody's business. In referring ethical decisions to a committee, there is a built-in potential for enervating the decision-making process by emphasizing secondary factors, such as economic concerns.

Third, the introduction of a review system for treatment of patients at the time of death could lead to a wider review system of all cases with cost control implications. The use of high technology in diagnosing patients' conditions could be subject to these committees also. In sum, then, it does not seem that placing jurisdictional review or decision-making powers in the hands of the ethics committee will lead to better treatment of people in danger of death.

However, it seems the ethics committee would be able to fulfill its purpose through educational functions alone. Formal health care education in the recent past has not prepared people for competent ethical decision making, and it does not look as if the situation will improve in the immediate future. The solution to this perceived lack of preparation, however, is not to put ethical decision making in the hands of a few. Rather, there should be "on-the-job" opportunities for health care professionals to assimilate the general and specific knowledge pertinent to ethical decision making. This can be done in a number of ways; through workshops, case studies, and consultation in individual cases, health care professionals can acquire the knowledge necessary for ethical decision making.

In addition, knowledge may be enhanced if the ethics committee outlines policies, to be approved and put into effect through the usual administrative process, for specific ethical problems. For example, several hospitals are formulating policies on withholding cardiopulmonary resuscitation. These policies do not remove the ethical responsibilities from the concerned persons; rather, they ensure more effective personal decision making because they set the limits within which such ethical decisions will be made.

CONCLUSION

Decisions concerning the care of people who are near death, whether they are old or newborn, involve many medical and ethical difficulties. There is no way to ensure that such decisions will be easy, but we can ensure that insofar as humanly possible such decisions will be well-informed and responsible and made with the benefit of the patient as the foremost and determining factor. We submit that given the history of health care and medicine, and given the tendency to impersonal decision making by committee process, all concerned will be better served if the responsibility for decision making rests with physicians, patients, and patients' families, rather than with an ethics committee.

45: Role of Ethics Committees

One of the first empirical studies of ethics committees in hospitals finds that ethics committees are used for everything from "acting as a public relations tool for justifying unpopular decisions resulting from discontinuing unprofitable services" to "serving as an alternative to the courts." Although most ethics committees have a more limited purview, the study revealed that many ethics committees believe they should be involved at some time in particular medical decisions concerning patient care.

In this essay, basing considerations on the nature of the physician-patient relationship, we discuss the responsibility for ethical decision making in medicine. The discussion attempts to set forth realistic guidelines for the activities of ethics committees.

THE PRINCIPLES

Physicians promise to help patients to avoid illness, to regain health, or to live with infirmity as vitally as possible. The objectives of the physician-patient relationship always presuppose that the physician will offer help in accord with the patient's personal values. Thus, medicine is not an abstract science dealing only with scientific principles to particular individuals. The social and spiritual dimensions of the persons to whom scientific principles are applied, as well as their varying desires and needs, make the inclusion of values a necessity in forming a medical plan. For this reason, Leon Kass maintains that medicine, by its very nature, is a "moral enterprise."[1]

In the recent past, some philosophers have maintained that in science one cannot progress logically from the "is" to the "ought," from the scientific to the ethical. Thus, they maintain, science and its applications are "value free"; the moral dimension of scientific and medical judgments is something added from other disciplines. If values are intrinsic to decisions concerning medical care, however, then there is no reason to say that a transition must be made from "is" to "ought." The "ought" or ethical dimension, is an integral part of the medical decision.

Physicians and patients (or proxies) both have something to contribute to the medical care decision. The patient or proxy primarily expresses the desires and values of the person seeking medical help. The physician mainly makes a diagnosis and designs a medical care program in accord with the expressed wishes of the patient. The medical care decision is a cooperative product based on mutual trust.

154

What role does medical ethics have in this description of medical decision making? Medical ethics is not a new subspecialty within medicine. Physicians, not ethicists or ethics committees, are responsible for ensuring that the ethical perspective is present in medical decisions. Maintaining that physicians decide one aspect of patient care and ethicists another is a caricature of both medicine and ethics. Ethicists are able to help physicians prepare for medical decision making in accord with the accepted ethical norms, but ethicists may never replace physicians. What are accepted ethical norms? Obtaining informed consent for therapy is an example of an accepted ethical norm for medical care. Ethicists help physicians understand the essential elements of informed consent but physicians ensure that informed consent is obtained.

Another accepted ethical norm of medical care states that physicians should not induce death but may allow patients to die in certain circumstances. Helping physicians understand the circumstances that allow them to apply this important but subtle norm is the role of the ethicist. Although a body of knowledge exists that justifies calling medical ethics a distinct discipline, and thus justifies the role of medical ethicists, there is no reason to make the medical ethicist a principal participant in medical decision making. In general, the medical ethicist acts as an educator and, in specific cases, as a consultant, which is simply a more personal form of education.

If we are to preserve the integrity of the physician-patient relationship, the ethics committee should be envisioned as a group of persons fulfilling the rule of the medical ethicist. Thus, they offer to health care professionals and their patients only education and consultation.

DISCUSSION

With this somewhat more specified function assigned to medical ethics and ethics committees, several observations are in order.

1. Ethics committees should devote intense activity to self-education. If the committee is to sponsor education and consultation according to accepted ethical principles, then the committee must be knowledgeable about the principles in question. Common sense does not suffice for sound ethical decisions. The President's Commission for the Study of Ethical Problems in Medicine and Biomedical and Behavioral Research has developed some principles for our pluralistic society. The Catholic Church, in accord with its notion of the nature of the human person, has also developed ethical norms for medical care. Depending on the character of the health care facility, the ethics committee should school itself in one or both sets of these principles.

2. The membership of the ethics committee need not include people "from all walks of life." When stating regulations for ethics committees, there

is a tendency to require membership of persons who are "nonscientific," who "represent the community," or who are "consumers of health care." Clearly, when membership of "outsiders" on ethics committees is recommended, there is a possibility that ethical decisions in medicine will be based on public opinion rather than on accepted ethical principles and the knowledge of medical practice. People from all walks of life may serve effectively on ethics committees in health care facilities if they are knowledgeable about ethics, but they do not qualify as ethical experts simply because they are "outside" the profession of health care. Rather, persons qualify for ethics committees through their ability to analyze issues from well-reasoned ethical perspectives.

3. The main purpose of ethics committees is to sponsor education programs for all persons associated with the health care facility. The formulation of policy in regard to ethical issues, such as policies for do-not-resuscitate (DNR) orders or transplantation of organs, simply represents more specific educational programs. If consultation on an ethical issue is requested by a physician or a patient (or proxy), the purpose should be to help the physician and/or patient to sort out their thinking. The ethics committee does not replace the physician or the patient. The concept that the ethics committee becomes some sort of jury before whom evidence is presented is a travesty of ethical decision making.

CONCLUSION

The foregoing vision of ethics committees does not call for a de-emphasis of these committees. True, if the relationship between the physician and the patient is to be respected, ethics committees will have a more limited responsibility than some would desire. However, the need for education in medical ethics should not be underemphasized. Physicians and other health care professionals do not know intuitively the principles of medical ethics. Thus, they require the input and expertise of the ethics committee in their ethical decision making.

NOTE

1. Leon Kass, *Toward a More Natural Science: Biology and Human Affairs* (New York, Free Press), 65.

46: Disregarding Patient Wishes: A Closer Look

Despite contemporary notions of patient autonomy and the emphasis on a patient's right to make health care decisions, treatment decisions are still made that disregard patient wishes. A survey of 1400 doctors and nurses indicated that a significant number of them "often violate their own personal beliefs and ignore requests from patients to withhold life support in cases of terminal illness." Moreover, they "often fail to provide adequate pain relief for dying patients in hospitals despite the patient's expressed wishes to be spared severe pain."[1] The extent of disregard for patients' wishes remains unknown. However, surveys and anecdotal evidence from health care workers substantiate the claim that such behavior inhibits proper care for dying patients. This essay will examine the causes of this disregard for patients' desires and propose a model of decision making that respects patient autonomy without absolutizing it to the detriment of both patient and society.

Four factors contribute to the neglect of patients' wishes at the end of life. First, some physicians and institutions fear legal reprisals and view overtreatment as the safest method of avoiding malpractice suits. Second, many health care professionals still perceive the patient's death as a sign of failure, both of themselves and of the vast array of life-sustaining technologies at their disposal. Third, health care personnel and institutions are sometimes unaware of ethical norms regarding the use or nonuse of life-sustaining treatments. Finally, health care professionals may believe that they know what is best for patients—even better than the patients themselves—ignoring in the process the particular life styles, attitudes, and values of patients. This is paternalism as understood in its classical sense.

PRINCIPLES

Resolving the problem of lack of respect for patients' requests must begin with an understanding of the appropriate role of patients in the health care decision-making process. Several reasons exist for asserting the importance of patients' perspectives in the decision-making process. First, each of us pursues various goals in life that help to fulfill us as human beings. Health must be considered as one of the principle goals we seek because good health affords us the opportunity to pursue many other goals and needs. Consequently, health is a matter of intense personal responsibility that necessarily requires the active agency of patients in the decision-making process. Second, treatment modalities cannot be considered abstractly. Treatments affect real people in real life situations, people who have differing value systems, needs, wants, and desires. Therefore, the patient's particular needs must be integrated into the decision-making process. The patient is best qualified to do this. Ultimately, the patient must live or die with the consequences of taking or not taking a treatment. Finally, our ability to choose is a constitutive part of our humanity. We are most human when we choose freely. The exercise of this freedom should be encouraged in health care in order to promote the dignity of the person. This is why autonomy is an important ethical principle. Of course, autonomy cannot be considered unbridled or interpreted in an overly individualistic sense. To do so would deny the fact that as individuals we exercise our freedom in a social and communal setting. Nevertheless, the patient's right to decide should in general be respected and promoted.

This understanding of ourselves suggests that neither paternalism nor unbridled autonomy offers an appropriate model of decision-making. Instead a shared decision-making process should be encouraged between the physician and patient. Doctors utilize their medical expertise and technical knowledge to offer potentially beneficial treatments to patients. Then, in light of their values and needs, patients reflect on the possible interventions and how they will impact on their lives. Together, physician and patients arrive at mutually beneficial decisions. Ultimately, this process works insofar as trust exists in the relationship. This trust engenders a spirit of dialogue that avoids the extremes of disregarding patients' wishes and unlimited autonomy.

DISCUSSION

Some proponents of a more pragmatic approach to decision making argue that a shared decision-making strategy should be pursued in an ideal world. But in the daily practice of medicine, rarely can idealistic concepts be actualized. However, the fruits of that "realistic" approach to medicine demands further examination in light of some recent trends in the world of health care. First, the growing emphasis on advance directives has developed in part out of a sense of distrust between patients and health care professionals. Patients have turned to written, legal documents to protect themselves from the unwanted assaults of technology at the end of life. Some physicians and institutions welcomed their introduction as a source of legal immunity from both patients and the government. Although today advance directives can serve a good purpose in promoting communication between the patient, family, and physician, their genesis partially resulted from a flaw in the patient-physician relationship. Second, the increasing clamor for legalized euthanasia and physician-assisted suicide reflects the pathological consequences of emphasizing the extremes of paternalism and autonomy. On one hand, the euthanasia movement in part indicates patient dissatisfaction with the disregard of their wishes, technological overtreatment, and under-utilization of pain medication. On the other hand, the movement also reflects an inappropriate understanding of patient autonomy wherein freedom is misunderstood to encompass whatever the patient desires, irrespective of the ethical and medical appropriateness of the patient's request. Third, the growth or at least perceived growth in recourse to malpractice suits presupposes an adversarial relationship between physician and patient. This trend was precipitated not so much by negligence or incompetence on the part of physicians but by an unwillingness to listen and communicate with patients and their families.[2] In sum, failing to consider input of patients has served only to escalate costs through overtreatment while simultaneously diminishing patients' well-being.

These recent trends, in conjunction with the fact that the surveyed health care professionals acted against their beliefs (what they knew in fact to be ethical), raise some serious concerns. To overcome this threat to the ethical provision of health care, several conceptual changes must occur. First, the ethical practice of medicine continues to be the best guarantee against legal liability. Overtreatment of the dying and overutilization of tests to avoid malpractice will do more to contribute to the problem than solve it because of the resulting erosion of the fiduciary or trusting relationship between physician and patient.

Second, the health care profession must reassess its understanding of death as an adversary and symbol of failure. Although we do not intentionally hasten a patient's death, death is a natural part of the process of life and should be accepted as such. Additionally, pain medication should be dispensed appropriately even though certain narcotics may result in an unintended hastening of the dying process.

Third, everyone in the decision-making process must continue to educate themselves about the ethical norms governing the appropriate use or nonuse of life sustaining treatments.

Fourth, and most important, physicians and nurses must acknowledge and respect the patient's right to refuse overly burdensome or ineffective treatments that serve only to prolong death rather than promote the goods of life. One grants that at times certain decisions by patients may be questioned if the patient's best interests are not being realized. Physicians are not merely technicians who follow a patient's requests blindly. Conflicted cases may require additional dialogue and even third-party mediation. However, those cases are considerably more infrequent than situations where the patient's best interests are compromised by actions that undermine appropriate patient autonomy.

CONCLUSION

A model of shared decision making between the doctor and patient offers a context in which ethical decisions about health care can be made. Today, certain patterns of behavior with regards to end of life decisions threaten to constrain the patient's ability to pursue legitimate goals in an appropriate fashion. Health care professionals must strive to eliminate unwarranted obstacles to healthy decision making. In the process of doing so, both patient and health care professional will benefit.

NOTES

1. Jane Brody, "Doctors Admit Ignoring Dying Patients' Wishes," *New York Times,* January 14, 1993. For the original data, see M. Solomon, et al., "Decisions Near the End of Life: Professional Views on Life-Sustaining Treatments," *American Journal of Public Health* 83 (1993): 14–23.

2. Gerald Hickson, et al., "Factors that Prompted Families to File Medical Malpractice Claims Following Perinatal Injuries," *JAMA* 267 (1992): 1359–63.

47: Genetics, Religion, and Ethics

Recently a conference was held in Houston, Texas, on "Genetics, Religion, and Ethics." Sponsored by the Institute of Religion and the Baylor College of Medicine, the conference sought to discuss the theological and ethical implications of the Human Genome project for medicine and public policy. The goal of the Human Genome Project is "to locate and describe the activity of human genes, to dispose for new treatments and cures for diseases, as well as to develop a deeper understanding of all biological processes."[1] Because the Human Genome project will influence the way we understand ourselves and will shape the practice of medicine, this essay will offer a synopsis of issues discussed, utilizing the threefold perspective of the conference in Houston.

1. *Genetic perspective*: The Human Genome Project sponsored and funded by the National Institutes of Health and the Department of Energy is well underway. The cost of the project will exceed 15 billion dollars over a period of 5 years. To date, progress has been impressive. Genes related to or causing specific genetic diseases have been identified. For example, the genes responsible for cystic fibrosis and myotonic dystrophy have been located. Researchers have cloned a gene involved in Fragile X Syndrome, thus allowing for more intensive study of the most common form of inherited mental retardation. To date, much of the information garnered concerns identification of genes that may cause defects if they do not function properly. Hence, the main benefit of the Genome Project has been more accurate and faster diagnosis of disease caused by genetic factors. Cure for most genetic defects is not available. But encouraging information in this regard was provided. A research project seeking to introduce a healthy gene into the DNA of a child whose immune system was functioning poorly seems to have been successful. The genetic defect, adenosine deaminase deficiency (ADA), causes severe combined immunodeficiency (SCID). While ADA defect is found in only about twenty-five children each year, the scientists conducting this research hope that the knowledge and experience gained in treating this disease will prove useful for treatment of several genetic disabilities such as cystic fibrosis, muscular dystrophy, or Down Syndrome. However, because the manner in which genetic defects occur and differ from one another,

161

applying technology that has been curative for one defect to another defect will be very difficult.[2]

2. *Ethical Perspective*: As might be expected, the application of knowledge derived from the Genome Project gives rise to several ethical issues. In private conversations, some participants questioned the wisdom of devoting so much money to the Genome Project when so many U.S. citizens lack access to adequate health care. The main ethical issues discussed publicly at the conference arise from distinctions between therapeutic and enhancement manipulation of genes and between somatic cell and germ cell manipulation. In regard to the first distinction, the following considerations are relevant. Therapeutic manipulation of genes seems to be acceptable and a natural outcome of the Genome Project. When defective genes are discovered, it is reasonable to seek methods to change the behavior of the genes in question, thus preventing or curing a serious handicap or pathology. However, the acceptance of enhancement manipulation is not so clear cut. Would it be beneficial if the human phenotype were altered through genetic manipulation so that a person were taller, slimmer, or more agile than she would be, given her natural genetic makeup? Even more radical, would it benefit a person if her genes that control aggression could be modified or muted? In principle, it would seem that enhancement changes would be ethically acceptable for a human person: (1) if they give support to human intelligence, and (2) if they did not suppress any of the fundamental human functions that integrate the human personality. Alteration in the human phenotype, which would make it impossible for human beings to experience the basic emotions, for example, would be detrimental because the emotional life is closely related to human intelligence and creativity. Again, alterations that would make human beings capable of reproduction only through in vitro fertilization would be antihuman. Any type of genetic engineering that involves "enhancement" should be undertaken only with the greatest caution. To put the matter in simple terms, we have a very difficult time planning effective traffic patterns in our cities or the collection and disposition of waste materials, let alone planning something as complicated as our genetic future.

The distinction between somatic cell and germ cell manipulation gives rise to the following considerations. Should the knowledge and therapy that results from the Genome Project be applied only to somatic cells, thus affecting one person at a time? Or may genetic therapy and/or genetic enhancement be directed toward germ cells, thus affecting the progeny of the person whose germ cells are manipulated? Most participants seemed to reject germ cell therapy, mainly because it is so difficult to predict how introducing one genetic alteration will affect other genes and how it would affect people generated in the future.

One disturbing issue in regard to genetic research as applied to prenatal diagnosis was not discussed publicly during the meeting. Because the discovery of genetic defects far exceeds the ability to cure, if a serious birth defect is discovered in prenatal screening, then it seems to be assumed that abortion of the infant is the only alternative and is ethically acceptable. Of course, the interpretation concerning what constitutes defective genes is very subjective. Surveys were cited in which 12 percent of prospective parents stated they would abort a baby whose genes indicated a future problem with obesity. Moreover, abortion as a means of sex selection is common in our society, even though some ethicists will decry it as a form of gender discrimination. In sum, there seems to be a supposition that every couple has the right to a perfect baby. If prenatal screening indicates that the infant does not "fit" the subjective desires of the parents, then abortion is accepted as an ethical alternative. While abortion of the unborn is a serious ethical issue at the personal level, an even more serious ethical issue arises at the social level. People assume that they have a right to a problem-free future and that human problems may be solved by eliminating human beings.

3. *Religious Perspective*: One of the speakers alluded to Dylan Thomas's poem, "A Child's Christmas in Wales" in which a young boy receives "books that told me everything about wasps, except why." Clearly, this sums up the Genome Project insofar as the religious or theological perspective is concerned. What will all this new information and the ability to eliminate many physical and mental defects teach us about being human; about the purpose of human life; about our ability to love God, ourselves, and other people? More specifically, what limits should we recognize as we acknowledge God's creative power?

While everyone at the conference was not happy with the term, the theological issues of genetic research and genetic manipulation seem to be summed up in the term "co-creator." As co-creators with God, what responsibilities and needs do we have to improve upon creation whether we are concerned with genetic manipulation of plants and animals or human beings? The following general norms seem to follow from the belief that human beings are created in the image and likeness of God and thus are responsible as co-creators for their own future: (a) God is a generous Creator, who in creating human beings also called them by the gift of intelligence to share in creative power. Consequently, God does not want human beings to leave fallow the talents that have been given them, but encourages them to improve on the universe; (b) such improvement is possible because theology can accept the idea that God has made an evolutionary universe in which the human race has been created through an evolutionary process that is not yet complete. Thus, God has called humankind to join in bringing the universe to its completion, and in doing this, God has not made them merely workers to execute orders or to add trifling original touches on their own. Rather, God has made them genuine co-workers and encourages them to exercise real creativity; and (c) human creativity depends on the human brain. Any alteration that would injure the brain and thus a person's creativity would indeed be a disastrous mutilation, especially if this were to be transmitted genetically, thus further polluting the gene pool with defects that might be hidden and incalculable.

Much of the information gained from the Genome Project will affect our bodies. But as often expressed during the conference, human beings are entities composed of body and spirit (soul). What affects our bodies will affect our spirit. Because we know our genetic makeup, we shall have a better notion of the factors that influence our behavior, but must we admit that genetic factors determine our behavior? As pointed out at the conference, the genetic difference between a chimpanzee and a human does not exceed 5 percent. But we know from faith and experience that humans are radically different from chimpanzees.

CONCLUSION

The ethical and theological issues arising from the Genome Project and the ability to manipulate somatic and germ cells will not go away. There is no "final solution." The importance of the information and technology resulting from the Genome Project and other genetic research cannot be overestimated. The changes in human life resulting from the Industrial Revolution will seem minor compared to the changes resulting from genetic research and technology. In order to avoid the misuse of genetic research and technology, constant vigilance and thoughtful reflection will be required.[3]

NOTES

1. Louis Sullivan, M.D. *The Genome Project*. Dept. of HHS, Wash. D.C., 1991, 1.

2. Inder Verma, "Gene Therapy," *Scientific American*, (November 1990), 68ff. (an excellent explanation of the means and methods of genetic manipulation).

3. cf. *Gene Watch*: A newsletter published by the Council for Responsible Genetics (CRG) seeking to alert the public to social and ethical issues raised by research and technology in human genetics.

48: Organ Donation: Priceless Gift or Market Commodity?

Over 2000 people die in the United States annually awaiting a suitable organ for transplantation. Moreover, every twenty minutes a new name is added to the list of people waiting for a kidney transplant. As the success of organ transplantation has increased, so has the demand for organs. Yet, the supply of donors has remained relatively constant over the past five years. Estimates vary, but only about 20 percent of potential cadaver donors actually end up being donors.[1] Recent efforts to maximize the retrieval of cadaveric organs have not succeeded. Required request laws that mandate that families of all potential donors be notified of the option to donate have been ineffective. Presumed consent, wherein it is presumed the person would want to donate one's organs unless specified otherwise, has been rejected as a viable alternative in the United States and has only met with limited success in Europe. In the United States, one untried solution to increase the supply of available organs is to create a market that provides incentives for donation. The buying and selling of organs initially strikes us as reprehensible and ghoulish on an emotional level. The National Organ Transplant Act of 1984 prohibits the acquisition, reception, and transfer of human organs for valuable consideration or payment as it affects interstate commerce laws. Several states have enacted similar legislation. However, is there a concomitant ethical basis for proscribing the element of financial compensation in the field of organ procurement?

LIVING DONORS

To facilitate the ethical analysis, one should divide the potential market into two types: a market for organs from living donors and one from cadavers (the purchase of fetal tissue and organs from induced abortion will not be considered here because of the intrinsic conflict of interest between the mother and the fetus). Recent stories from Latin America and India where the poor sell kidneys to rich transplant recipients have aroused moral outrage and condemnations of exploitation. Yet, justifications for such behavior are frequently offered. First, supply is increased. Second, the donors receive compensation for their organs which can sometimes be an economic lifesaver. Third, autonomy is enhanced as individuals exercise their liberty to use and dispose of their bodies as they see fit. Finally, people sell blood and other bodily products, so why not organs?

165

The first two arguments are strictly consequentialist in nature. The merits of such arguments are debated on an empirical basis. The commercialization of organ procurement may result in a net decrease of available organs because it may further suspicion of the transplant field. Also, those who would give altruistically would be offended by the commercialization of the "gift of life." But even if supply would increase, would such good ends justify the means to them? Is there something inherently problematic with this type of practice? The sale of organs appears to be an act of financial desperation by the poor. The money offered as an enticement to donate is so coercive that it influences the individual unduly. This precludes the possibility of obtaining informed consent. Freedom is so compromised in such a case that true consent is not possible.

One might argue that financial gain coerces the poor into accepting more hazardous jobs. We do not prevent the poor from accepting such risky jobs; why should we prohibit the removal of kidneys if it does not pose too great a risk? Two distinctions might be helpful. First, people have the freedom to leave a job at any time whereas the removal of a kidney is a permanent procedure. Second, although work cannot be reduced to a transaction because it also pertains to an essential aspect of fulfillment for the human person, there is an inherently appropriate connection between work and just compensation for services rendered. To apply such an analogy to organ donation reduces the person to a commodity, to a property composed of various body parts. Courtney Campbell comments that to reduce ourselves to this "expresses estrangement from our embodied experience."[2] We not only have stewardship over our bodies, but we also "are our bodies." This is why the selling of blood products does not repulse us whereas the selling of organs does. Traditionally, people have argued that one can sell blood products because the sale presents no risks and the blood is a renewable source whereas organs are not. But, the issue goes much deeper. When we sell the pint of blood, we do not perceive the body as being affected. However, when an organ is removed, one knows that one's body is being affected. Thus, the only acceptable motivation for live donation has been charity. Whereas the selling of body parts for money alienates us from ourselves, altruistic donation reaches deeply into the meaning of personhood. As creatures directed to share our love, organ donation fulfills that desire to be charitable. This is why we perceive the selling of organs as being reprehensible while charitable donation is seen as courageous and magnanimous.

CADAVER SOURCES OF ORGANS

Can the same reasoning be applied to the case of cadaveric sources of organs? In the case of cadaver donation, the previous problems of risk, coercion, and the lack of consent are conspicuously absent. As a result, a more concerted effort to introduce financial inducements has been adopted. Could a market mechanism be established that is neither offensive nor easily abused? Most would agree that it seems callous, offensive, and grossly utilitarian to come to the grieving survivors and offer direct payment for their loved one's organs. The body is not distinct from the person and to treat the body so blatantly as a commodity, as a collection of parts, offends the memory of the person. However, could more subtle and indirect forms of remuneration be more acceptable and less offensive? Indirect market methods of compensation might include: paying for funeral costs for the family, offering a type of life insurance program where beneficiaries would be reimbursed after donation, reducing health insurance premiums, waiving driver's license fees in exchange for signing the donor card, and even creating a futures market. Proponents argue that creating such incentives to promote donation benefits all. The corpse would not be harmed. Needy individuals will receive organs. People will receive compensation. In fact, not to do this would seem unethical because many are condemned to death because of the lack of organs. Naturally, it would be better for people to give out of pure altruism. But if such is not the case, why not provide an incentive?

Various arguments are offered in response to such reasoning. From a practical standpoint, such an approach again may be counterproductive because it will decrease altruistic donation. Additionally, payment for organs will increase the cost of an already expensive technology especially if an open market would develop. Finally, minorities and the poor may be further alienated from the system because they feel they are being paid to provide organs for the rich. On the more symbolic level, even after death, a transcendent relationship remains between the person and the body. The corpse is not just decaying matter or property. Although our language sometimes refers to the body as property, especially in law, one should not assume that a similar terminology is philosophically appropriate. Relatives do not own the body of the deceased as if it were property or even quasi-property. Rather, they exercise respectful and dignified stewardship over the body because of the intrinsic link to the person and the obligations due that person as a member of the human community. Admittedly, the buying of cadaver organs does not harm the deceased *per se*. However, there may be considerable potential for harm to the human community by undermining its sense of altruism and compassion. By moving away from the concept of organ donation as gift, one transforms the body and ultimately the person into commodity and property. The more market oriented the inducement strategy, the greater will be the assault to the dignity of the person. The general public's apprehension of the commercialization of organ donation should not be ignored. Although sometimes dismissed as inexact and nebulous, this intuitional moral sense that operates in the realm of symbol can arouse the conscience and direct us to the moral good.

CONCLUSION

The buying and selling of organs from living donors seems inappropriate. It is not absolutely clear that providing subtle financial inducements like helping to pay funeral expenses in exchange for cadaveric organs is intrinsically wrong, but the consequences of such an approach may not have the desired effects and may distort our vision of the human person. Given the gravity of the issue and the lives at stake, further discussion needs to occur in the area of cadaveric donation to clarify our understandings of life and death, body and property. Is "gift" the only paradigm in which to understand organ donation? Or can one conceptually juxtapose self-centered and altruistic motivations in the same action? If over 70 percent of U.S. citizens believe in donation, before giving further consideration to the sale of cadaver organs, other alternatives should be exhausted. For example, reexamining the concept of presumed consent and encouraging compliance with required request laws by means of additional education and training may help. Unfortunately, the numbers indicate that supply may never meet demand. Therefore, we may need to deal with the harder question of reducing demand rather than increasing supply. Ultimately, will we have to reassess the technology in light of all of the other important goods of health care that remain unfulfilled today?

NOTES

1. There are about 4,500 actual organ donors from 20–25,000 deaths from which organs could be procured. R.W. Evans, et al. suggest the number of potential donors may be at most 11,000. See "The Potential Supply of Organ Donors: An Assessment of the Efficacy of Organ Procurement Efforts in the United States," *JAMA* 267 (1992): 239–46.

2. C. Campbell, "Body, Self, and the Paradigm of Property," *Hastings Center Report* 22 (Sept-Oct, 1992):42.

49: AIDS Research: Innovative Methods

Recent developments in the testing of drugs for AIDS patients portend significant changes in the way clinical trials will be conducted in the United States. The developments and changes in question give rise to serious ethical issues. Traditionally, the standard procedure for testing drugs requires clinical trials in which one group of people, the control group, receives placebos, (or the standard treatment), and another group of people receives the drug being tested. In order to avoid the "placebo effect," participants in the trial do not know whether or not they are receiving the placebo (or standard treatment) or the drug being tested. If the researcher working with the participant of the study is also unaware of the substance the subjects receive, this type of research is known as a double-blind study.

In addition, new drugs are not approved for public use until three series of clinical trials are conducted. The first trial tests the safety of the substance—does any serious harm befall the first people to receive the drug? The second test is for effectiveness—does the new drug combat the illness or disease in question? The third trial investigates side effects—what unwanted symptoms result from varying doses of the drug?

The aforementioned methods were followed in the first clinical trials testing drugs for the alleviation of AIDS. But the recent response of AIDS activists to traditional clinical trials has hampered drug trials and called into question ethical principles upon which they are based.[1] In some cases patients in the clinical trial have had their pills tested. If they are receiving the placebo or a treatment they consider unsatisfactory, they drop out of the trial. Fewer and fewer AIDS patients are willing to volunteer for clinical trials, stating that they do not wish to be guinea pigs for science. Moreover, AIDS activists are calling for a faster method of making new drugs available and demanding that they be made available to more people, maintaining that persons in danger of death will not be concerned about stringent safety standards.

In order to improve the situation of AIDS patients, AIDS activists are demanding of the federal agencies that clinical trials be considered as primarily therapeutic; that all patients in a clinical trial be given the drug being tested; and that experimental drugs be released to any patient who wishes to use them. Not only has the request been made for agencies of the federal government to change their policies for testing drugs, several physicians and people affected with AIDS have initiated private studies of drugs that might alleviate AIDS

169

without observing the research safeguards. Unlike government-funded clinical trials, the private studies are not overseen by impartial committees (IRB), which analyze risk, benefit, and informed consent in order to protect subjects from being harmed by research. Clearly, the demands of AIDS patients and their proponents challenge the usual way of conducting research in the scientific community.

PRINCIPLES

The ethical questions underlying the request of the AIDS activists to change the method of testing drugs are:

1. What is the purpose of clinical trials? Should they be designed to acquire scientific knowledge, or should they be structured, in order to deliver therapy? For years, clinical trials were considered first and foremost as research projects, that is, the primary purpose was to discover knowledge that would benefit the human community. If the subjects of the protocol would receive some therapeutic benefit in the course of the trial, well and good. But the clinical trial would be designed in such a way as to ensure that the desire for therapeutic benefit for the subject would not endanger the discovery of knowledge. In clinical trials for cancer drugs for example, the subjects are often limited to those who are seriously ill; and while there is a remote chance that the drug being tested may be of some help to the subjects, the clinical trial is not designed to be primarily therapeutic.

2. What is needed to ensure informed consent on the part of a person participating in a clinical trial? Briefly, the person participating in a clinical trial should be aware of the goals, procedures, risks, and benefits of the research project and should have these goals, procedures, risks, and benefits explained in his or her own language. Finally, the subject should make a free decision; hence, coercing one to participate in a clinical trial is unethical. If these norms are observed, then one may assent ethically to participate in the trial.

DISCUSSION

From an ethical perspective, how evaluate the requests of the AIDS activists? First of all, no matter what the purpose of a clinical trial, the well-being of the participants must be the foremost concern of those who design the protocol. Even if the principal purpose is to obtain scientific knowledge, the risks to the subject must be proportionate to the benefits derived from the trial. Though people with AIDS may indeed be desperate, researchers are not allowed to expose them to totally unknown risks. Private trials that do not evaluate the safety of the drug in question before distributing it to people even if these people may die as a result of AIDS, would seem to be unethical.

Secondly, it does seem unfair to ask AIDS victims to join a clinical trial in which they may receive a placebo instead of a drug that may improve their condition. When the clinical trials for AZT were conducted, they were evaluated by computing the number of AIDS patients who died in the group that received AZT compared to the number of those who died in the group that received the placebo. Would it have been possible to give all participants in the trial the drug being tested and then compare their physical condition and longevity with results predicted from experience with AIDS patients in the past? Or, could a factor short of death be utilized for measuring the efficiency of the drug, making the test more flexible and open to more people? Certainly the scientific knowledge gained from a test in which all receive the drug being tested would not be as easily acquired nor as conclusive as knowledge gained from the traditional double-blind clinical trial. But is it not possible to design trials in which the goal of therapy is more prominent, even though scientific knowledge remains the principal goal?

While a double-blind study is ethically acceptable if the subject understands the essential elements of the study and freely commits to participation in the study, the need for such studies may not be as great in the future. As a result of objections from AIDS activists, the Biostatistics Research Committee at the NIH is using computers to design clinical trials that will produce statistically valid data without using placebos.

CONCLUSION

The federal agencies in charge of drug research have responded favorably to the requests of the AIDS activists. Whatever the innovations and changes being initiated in the clinical trials for drugs that will combat AIDS, one ethical principle should remain paramount. The most unethical type of trial is one that does not yield a reliable answer. Hence, as clinical trials become more therapeutic, the need to acquire certain scientific knowledge must not be forgotten.

NOTE

1. News and Comments: "AIDS Drug Trials Enter New Age," *Science*, Oct. 6, 1989, p. 19.

50: Human Research with Animals

In the last century, a movement to limit the use of animals in medical research began in England. Led by Frances Power Cobbe (1822–1904), the movement opposed vivisection of animals, a term used to signify opposition to the use of animals, especially living animals, in any form of research. In response to the importuning of several prominent citizens who supported the movement, Parliament in 1876 passed the Cruelty to Animals Act, which required the registration of places where experiments were performed on living animals and required licensing of researchers and permission for particular types of research. British antivivisectionists are still active and have had the regulations on animal research strengthened by subsequent laws in 1913 and 1965. Not surprisingly, the movement spread to the United States, resulting in federal legislation setting limits and regulations on research with animals (1966). But significant limitations of animal research have also resulted from organized volunteer organizations such as ISAP (Institute for Study of Animal Problems) and FRAME (Fund for the Replacement of Animals in Medical Experiments). These organizations work openly in the public forum and promote their objectives through publicity and political action. In addition to these more or less irenic groups, there are more vehement organizations such as PETA (People for Ethical Treatment of Animals) and ALF (Animal Liberation Front), which approve of direct attacks upon research facilities. These groups seem to think any action they perform to prevent research on animals is justified because they feel so strongly about it and people start to listen if you destroy property.

Many people are not against using tissue from dead animals for research, but seek to eliminate research upon living animals. For others, putting animals to death in order to use them in research presents a problem. Proponents of this position argue that animal research is not necessary. Many research projects using animals are ephemeral. For example, they assert that most experiments using living animals are not used for "medical" experiments but rather to test such nonessential items as cosmetics, shampoo, and food coloring. Finally, they maintain that computers could replace animals in most research projects. Researchers dispute this latter assertion pointing out that in the past forty years, vaccine research, which has led to vaccines for polio, diphtheria, measles, mumps, whooping cough, and rubella, could never have been developed through computer models.

172

MOVEMENT'S STAYING POWER

What gives the antivivisectionist movement such staying power? Most of the anticruelty societies started in the last century have long since disbanded. But while the antivivisectionist movement has been less than popular in some areas of the United States, it never dies out. Indeed, it seems to be increasing in numbers in the latter part of this century. There seems to be a number of reasons that attract people to the movement. First of all, some people desire to protect animals from pain. As Jeremy Bentham stated in the eighteenth century: "The question is not can they reason, nor can they talk, but, can they suffer?" One response to this aphorism is to distinguish between pain and suffering. While animals may experience pain, it is an instinctive reaction and does not connote true suffering, which requires the power of reflection as well as sense cognition.

Second, some adhere to the movement because they maintain that animals are not a different species from human beings and should not be considered "at the disposal of human beings." Animals as well as humans, they maintain, should be protected from painful experiences because there is basically no difference between these two species of living beings. One spokesperson for this philosophy even maintains that there would be no difference between using retarded children instead of animals for research, even lethal research. Whether this theory, which equates animals and humans, is a cause or an effect of the antivivisectionist movement is not clear, but it seems that the movement existed long before this philosophical underpinning was developed. At any rate, until such time as dogs and horses organize anticruelty societies in favor of their owners and masters, the argument equating animals and humans will remain in the realm of pure theory.

Another factor that enables the movement to survive is the heavily publicized "abuses" in animal research. For example, in the early 80s a center specializing in simian research was accused of keeping the apes and monkeys in filthy quarters. Also in the early 80s, dogs were shot and wounded to enable military doctors to practice sewing gunshot wounds caused by a new type of ammunition. Both events led to an outcry by the well-organized animal rights societies and then by the general public. Court proceedings in response to the charges against the research scientists in the simian project show than an animal rights activist infiltrated the project. While other researchers were on vacation, he allowed conditions in the laboratory to deteriorate, and then took pictures depicting "unsanitary conditions." Investigation of the wound healing project revealed the dogs were anesthetized before the research began and did not endure pain.

While these aforementioned theories and happenings give impetus to the movement, it seems there is another influence underlying the longevity of the movement. This factor is seldom mentioned in studies in favor of or against animal research. This unmentioned factor is a feeling of mistrust that many people have for science, technology, and scientists. From mistrust develops the attendant feeling that "all would be all right again" if we could only put science and technology back in the bottle. Because the general public apprehends scientists as engaged in occupations that are far removed from ordinary activities of daily life, they are prone to mistrust them and blame the shortcomings of technology upon them. It is easy to depict scientists as using animals in a harmful manner because the ordinary person does not see the intimate connection between animal research and improved human health.

TOWARD A SOLUTION

Considering the distance between scientists and the general population, it will be difficult to convince people of the value of animal research unless they realize the personal benefits that accrue from such protocols. With this in mind, several physicians and scientists have organized a national group called The Incurable Ill for Animal Research (IIFAR) with the slogan: "Lab animals save human lives and animal lives." The thrust of the organization's literature directly ties animal research to the future cure or alleviation of some of the more fatal and debilitating diseases that afflict young and old in our country, such as cystic fibrosis, leukemia, and diabetes. Even with the formation of IIFAR the antivivisectionists out-spend by a wide margin those who see benefit to human life resulting from animal research.

The fundamental reason that justifies the use of animals in the quest for a better life for human beings is found in the relationship of humans to animals. Human beings demean themselves if they abuse animals. But in the effort to prolong life, to improve health, and to foster the overall well-being of society, humans have a moral need and legal right to use animals just as they have the need and right to use minerals and plants for the same purposes. This is the common sense teaching upon which progress in culture and civilization are based. Moreover, it is also the teaching of religions that seek to improve the human condition by recognizing that beings with spiritual faculties have the responsibility to act as stewards over other created beings.

51: Euthanasia: On the Horizon?

"Movement to legalize euthanasia could succeed in the near future." This is the lead headline in a newsletter on medical ethics. For centuries, physicians and others in health care have been dedicated to protecting and preserving life. If the effort to have euthanasia accepted succeeds, physicians and others in health care would be expected to cause death. Participation in euthanasia would not only pervert the purpose of health care, it would also destroy all trust and confidence on the part of patients. With this potential damage in mind, a closer look at euthanasia and the factors disposing people to accept it is in order.

PRINCIPLES

The term euthanasia comes from Greek words that mean "good death." In common parlance, euthanasia implies that a stronger person causes the death of a weaker, suffering, or debilitated person. From an ethical perspective the elements involved in euthanasia are the intention of the person acting (the agent) and the results of the effect of the agent's action. The effect of the intention to perform euthanasia may be achieved by placing an act or by withholding an act. Examples of euthanasia accomplished through placing an act would be injecting poison into a sick person's system or smothering a suffering person with a pillow. But euthanasia may also be accomplished by withholding a life-prolonging action; for example, by withholding food from a debilitated patient when there are medical indications that food will help the person recover from his illness.

To signify the difference between euthanasia that is accomplished through an act, and euthanasia that is accomplished by omitting an act, a distinction is often made between active and passive euthanasia. The impression is conveyed that while active euthanasia is ethically unacceptable, passive euthanasia is acceptable because it does not require a positive action that brings about death. From an ethical perspective, the distinction between active and passive euthanasia is meaningless. If the intention of the agent is to cause the death of a patient, then an unethical effect results whether by means of placing an action or withholding an action.

If euthanasia is unethical, must the life of every suffering and comatose person be prolonged as long as possible? By no means. If a person has a fatal pathology, an ethical decision must be made whether to circumvent or alleviate the fatal pathology. The decision concerning the use of therapy should be made by the patient if he or she is competent, by a proxy if the patient is incompetent. The physician and other health care professionals supply the necessary information for an informed decision on the part of the patient or proxy. The criteria for withholding or discontinuing therapy when a fatal pathology is present are twofold: whether the therapy is effective for prolonging life, and whether the therapy would cause excessive burden in relation to the anticipated benefit. If one or the other criteria applies, then the therapy need not be utilized or, if already begun, may be discontinued. In such circumstances, the intention of the agent is not to cause the patient's death. Rather, if the therapy is deemed ineffective to prolong life, then the intention of the agent is simply to avoid doing something useless or futile; always an ethical imperative. If the therapy is deemed excessively burdensome in relation to the benefit for the patient, then the intention of the person removing or withholding therapy is to remove a burden from the patient. Clearly, when effectiveness of therapy is being evaluated, the physician will have more responsibilities than when burden and benefit are being evaluated.

The distinction between euthanasia and "allowing a patient to die" is often misunderstood. Some people maintain that this distinction splits hairs. But in reality, there is a great difference between the two actions. First of all, the intention of the two actions are entirely different. Second, in euthanasia, the intention brings about death by prompting the performance or withholding of an act. Allowing a person with a fatal pathology to die when there is no ethical obligation to prolong life does not cause death directly. Rather, the person dies because of the fatal pathology, which has not been circumvented or alleviated. In both cases death ensues: in euthanasia death is directly intended by the agent and is accomplished by a positive act or by withholding care that is ethically required. In "allowing to die," on the other hand, death is the unwanted side effect of a good ethical action.

DISCUSSION

Why is there a growing trend toward accepting euthanasia in our society? Briefly, let us mention some of the more prominent reasons:

1. Ronald Cranford, M.D., a leading expert in the case of comatose patients, maintains that the practices of the medical profession are fueling the drive toward euthanasia. The customs of medical care lead physicians to utilize all life-support systems without asking the proper ethical questions: Is the therapy effective for prolonging life? Does the therapy in question cause an excessive burden for the patient?
2. Another cause of the trend toward euthanasia is the practice of prolonging physiological function when it has been determined medically that cognitive-affective function cannot be restored. Specifically,

health care professionals must question when the therapy to prolong life is truly effective. In the face of medical and hospital opposition, the courts of several states have maintained that life-sustaining mechanisms are not ethically nor legally required if only physiological function can be sustained.

3. When considering excessive burden, many people will recognize only physiological burden (physical pain and suffering) as a reason for removing life-support therapy. But psychological, social, and spiritual burden should be considered as well. Considering the social burden to the patient requires that the burden to the family must be considered as well.

4. Another attitude leading people to promote euthanasia is the desire to be "in control of one's life." However, as the psychiatrist, David Peretz points out: "The desire to be in complete control of one's life is irrational and unhealthy; we are not masters of our fate in regard to many important events in our lives."[1]

CONCLUSION

The foregoing seem to be more prominent reasons for the trend in our society to accept euthanasia as an acceptable method of terminating life. It seems that each factor results from an inaccurate ethical evaluation either of the purpose of life or the purpose of medical care.

NOTE

1. David Peretz, "The Illusion of Rational Suicide," *Hastings Center Report*, 11 (1981): 40.

52: Suicide: A Rational Choice?

When discussing ethical issues surrounding suicide, our main question is not, "Should people who commit suicide be criticized?" Experience and intuition demonstrate that most persons who take their own lives do so because they are emotionally disturbed and act compulsively. Thus, their freedom of choice is greatly restricted or nonexistent. Too many of us know dear friends or family members whose suicidal deaths demonstrate the lack of psychological freedom. Indeed, many experts in suicidology today seem to take it for granted that all suicides are compulsive and irrational. Our question in this essay then concerns the contemporary tendency to present suicide as "a rational choice," that is, to present it as the best manner to die in some circumstances.

PRINCIPLES

Among the ancient Greeks and Romans, suicide was both condemned and defended, as it also was in Eastern cultures. The Epicureans, who considered pleasure and peace of mind the highest good, argued that it was better to kill oneself than endure life if it had become more painful than pleasurable or peaceful. The Stoics, who believed that rigid self-control was the highest good, argued that it was permissible to kill oneself if suffering or torture might force one to lose self-control. Dualists taught that the soul, which is the real person, is burdened by the body in this life; hence suicide might be justified as a laying down of this burden. Even today, some believe it ethical to choose suicide for the sake of honor. Recently some Irish and Vietnamese chose suicide by self-starvation and self-immolation to protest injustice and oppression.

The monotheistic religions of Judaism, Christianity, and Islam have always opposed suicide because they regard life as God's gift, which people must use not as owners but as faithful stewards. Consequently, we cannot escape accounting to God for our stewardship of this one life given on earth, nor can we reject the body, which will always be part of us. This view was anticipated by Plato, who argued that suicide is a rejection of our responsibility to self, to the community of which one is a part, and to God who gave life. In a different way, another philosopher, Immanuel Kant, argued that suicide is the greatest of crimes because it is a person's rejection of morality itself, since a human being must be his or her own moral lawgiver. Committing suicide means treating oneself as a thing (means) rather than as a person (an end in oneself). In sum, in theological and philosophical reasoning, suicide has been considered for centuries as an unethical act, even though responsibility was seldom imputed to the unfortunate persons who performed the action.

DISCUSSION

Today, however, this classic stand expressed in the monotheistic religions is being called into question. In the United States and England, societies exist that promote suicide as an ethical action, a "rational" alternative to life, especially if a person is beset by depression, loneliness, severe infirmity, or serious suffering. Usually the reasons put forward for approving suicide as an ethical choice are that people should have the right to be autonomous and to control their own destiny or that people should not have to suffer pain, loneliness, or degradation at the time of death. Although these are professed reasons for the modern reexamination of the traditional stance, a noted psychiatrist and suicidologist, David Peretz, sees a more subtle cause for this change of thought:

> Under the unprecedented stress of recent decades, denial mechanisms are breaking down and we have become increasingly vulnerable to the threats of intensely painful feelings of anxiety, fear, panic, rage, guilt, shame, grief, longing and helplessness. In order to avoid being overwhelmed, we seek new ways to adapt. . . .I believe that the growing concern with a good death, death with dignity and the right-to-die reflect this search . . . If our deepest known fear is of being destroyed, and we cannot deal with that fear, we take refuge in planning death and rational suicide. We find comfort in the illusion, "It will not be done to me. . . . I will do it myself.[1]

Peretz feels this is a dangerous motivation because it fosters the harmful illusion of personal omnipotence.

Two other unrealistic and therefore unethical elements are involved in rational suicide. First, the call for rational suicide is based on the notion that personal autonomy or independence is the goal of human life. Rational suicide says: If one cannot be autonomous or independent, then life is not worth living. This is simply one more expression of radical individualism, a philosophy that weakens human community and places little value on social justice. Both experience and wisdom demonstrate, however, that interdependence, not independence, is the goal of human life. To admit that one is weak and needs help is not a denial or a perversion of one's humanity. Rather, accepting help is a means to fulfill one's humanity. The weak and suffering offer an opportunity to others to fulfill their humanity by responding with care and kindness. The perfectly autonomous person would not need other people; can one imagine a more boring and self-centered individual?

A second unethical element in rational suicide is that it mythologizes the act of self-destruction. To mythologize something is to give it powers it does not possess. Rational suicide presents self-destruction as a problem-free solution to the very serious human problems of physical suffering, loneliness, severe depression, or infirm old age. But we do not eliminate human problems by eliminating human beings. Rather, we eliminate or alleviate human problems through compassion, care, and loving concern. The problems that rational suicide would pretend to eliminate are often problems with which individuals learn to live through the help of caring relatives or friends.

CONCLUSION

The present-day emphasis on the right-to-die and death with dignity may blind us to the right to life of the weak, infirm, and aged. The cost of combating the human problems of loneliness, infirmity, and depression is not self-destruction; rather, it is the development of a compassionate, caring, and generous community. Although not simple, this is a development rather than a perversion of our humanity.

NOTE

1. David Peretz, "The Illusion of Rational Suicide," *Hastings Center Report* 11 (1981): 40–42.

53: Aid in Dying: The Myth of "Managed Death"

A few years ago, voters in the state of Washington defeated an initiative that proposed to legalize active euthanasia and assisted suicide. Had the initiative passed, conscious and competent patients in terminal conditions, having less than six months to live, could have requested and received "aid in dying" from their physicians. Proponents of active euthanasia and assisted suicide argued that medicalized killing is the final and appropriate caring intervention of the physician in the life of a patient. Moreover, this "aid in dying" allows patients and physicians to manage death, thereby "taking responsibility for our technology, by assuring people who are its subjects that they will not be crucified on a cross of steel operating tables, shunts and tubes."[1]

Many opponents of the initiative held that concerns about the sanctity and inviolability of human life were enough to demonstrate the wrongness of the proposals. Others argued that, even if there may be some justification for responding to the request for assistance when the competent patient asks to be killed, legalizing such practices would place society and the medical profession at the peak of the well-worn slippery slope. In no time, they argued we would be euthanizing the incompetent and the elderly in an attempt to bring health care costs under control or for some other less noble reason. Still others maintained that society should neither ask nor allow its physicians to do things that might undermine the trust we place in them by engaging in actions that are inconsistent with the identity of "physician as healer."

The debate raised by proposals to legalize euthanasia and assisted suicide too often is carried on in a context of confusion. This confusion results in a lack of clarity about what euthanasia and assisted suicide mean and involve. For example, many incorrectly include under the broad category of "euthanasia" not only killing upon request but also removal of useless or excessively burdensome life support as well as provision of adequate pain relief that may hasten death as a secondary effect. In addition, because the discussion of euthanasia and assisted suicide often begins with claims about a right to die, many conclude that the ethical issue is simply one of responding to the requests of autonomous patients. When framed in this way, the issues are interpreted almost exclusively in terms of questions about control. How can the suffering or dying patient maintain some semblance of control in what many argue is a situation that inevitably "robs the person of dignity?" By concluding that "I will do it to myself, before it is done to me."[2]

CLARIFYING THE ISSUES

In order to assess ethically proposals for legalized euthanasia and assisted suicide, it is necessary to define terms and clarify the confusions noted above. Accordingly, suicide is a voluntary act by which one intends and causes one's own death. Suicide can be accomplished by acts of commission (e.g., shooting oneself) or by acts of omission (e.g., starving oneself to death). What is common to both is the introduction of a cause of death. Assisted suicide implies that the person cannot accomplish the intention and/or action to bring death about alone. Assistance in the suicide of another can be accomplished by acts of commission (e.g., prescribing a lethal dose of medication and instructing the person in its use). Assistance also can be rendered in a more passive way through persuasion and encouragement. In either case, the person who contributes to the death-dealing effort shares in the intention to bring death about through the introduction of a causative agent.

Second, euthanasia, whether active or passive, is an act or an omission that of itself or by intention causes death. Euthanasia can be accomplished by actively introducing a cause of death not already present (e.g., death by lethal injection) or by failing to circumvent the deadly effects of a cause already present when there is a duty to do so (e.g., withholding antibiotics to treat pneumonia in a child with Down's Syndrome *because* of the Down's Syndrome).

Third, both assisted suicide and euthanasia are clearly distinct from the ethical decision to withhold or withdraw ineffective or seriously burdensome life-prolonging therapies. When life is threatened by a condition internal to the person, that is by a fatal pathology, the cause of death is already present. If life-prolonging therapies can offer the patient no benefit, their removal is not a decision to kill the patient. Rather, it is a decision to forgo interventions that are ineffective or that impose serious burden. Although in such circumstances death may be welcomed as a release from suffering, it is neither intended nor caused as a means to overcome suffering.

Finally, proposals to respond to suffering by offering a "managed death" simply means that the one who suffers is eliminated. Such a response insures neither control over the dying process nor does it enhance the dignity of the one who suffers. In the Netherlands, physicians are protected from criminal prosecution if they respond to the request of patients for assisted death providing they meet several criteria. One such criterion is that there must be suffering that the person describes as intolerable. Many Dutch physicians claim that most if not all physical pain can be controlled by the judicious use of medication. Thus, the kind of suffering that leads most terminally ill patients in the Netherlands to request active euthanasia is emotional or psychological suffering, that is, suffering "dependent on subjective elements that often cannot be addressed effectively."[3]

However, since Elizabeth Kubler-Ross did her ground-breaking work with the dying, we have known a good deal about the content of the psychological suffering that terminally ill persons experience. They suffer from fear of the unknown that naturally accompanies the dying process. They suffer from the fear of becoming a burden on families and loved ones as they become less able to care for themselves. They suffer from the fear of being isolated from others by an experience that can only be understood fully by the one having it. And they suffer from fear of being abandoned by family, friends, and care givers. Certainly, these forms of suffering pose significant challenges to care givers. But the hospice experience has taught us that the willingness to accompany the dying person on the journey toward death goes a long way toward addressing these deeper levels of suffering. Hospice has also shown us that physical suffering can be managed by commitment to provide adequate and appropriate pain relief. Finally, hospice programs reassure patients and families that, while sophisticated technologies that can only prolong the dying process will not be used in the final days of life, other forms of appropriate care will be provided and the dying person will not be abandoned.

CONCLUSION

The question to be answered, then, is this: Is "aid in dying" or managed death an ethically appropriate response to the needs and suffering of the terminally ill? Although some may disagree, the common moral vision in western society consistently has answered "no" to this question. The basis for this response is the conviction that certain kinds of intentions and the actions to accomplish them are beyond the authority of human agents. The killing of innocent human beings by one's own volition not only inflicts harm on the one killed but harms society as well. Killing actions do nothing to address the realities that cause suffering for terminally ill persons. Legalizing such actions only ensures that less effort will be expended by care givers and others in the future in attempting to respond appropriately to the needs of the dying.

NOTES

1. David C. Thomasma & Glenn C. Graber, *Euthanasia: Toward an Ethics Social Policy* (New York: Continuum, 1990), 6.
2. David Peretz, "The Illusion of Rational Suicide," *The Hastings Center Report*, 11 (1981): 41.
3. Pieter Admiraal, M.D., "A Physician's Responsibility to Help a Patient Die." Presentation given at Controversies in the Care of the Dying Patient, February 14–16, 1991, Orlando, FL.

54: Proposition 161: Dying with Dignity in California

A few years ago, voters in California defeated a bill that would have allowed mentally competent, terminally ill adults to request and receive physician aid in dying. Had the bill passed, qualified persons would have been allowed to execute an advance directive to require a willing physician to end life in a "painless, humane, and dignified manner." Physicians complying with such a directive were assured of protection from civil and criminal liability as were other participating health care professionals and institutions. Proponents of this legislation argued that adequate safeguards have been written into the bill to avoid any potential abuses that might occur.[1]

This is the second such proposal to have been defeated in the past few years. Underlying this and similar proposals is the expressed concern that the rights of chronically and terminally ill patients are not protected adequately by current state laws. Proponents of this legislation argue that persons with terminal illness should be guaranteed the right to exercise the "most basic of freedoms," i.e., self-determination. By determining the time and manner of one's own death, it is argued, individuals can eliminate the pain and suffering associated with debilitating, terminal illness and can, in this way, maintain their dignity. Several other states have similar proposals that will be placed before voters in coming elections. While we cannot anticipate the outcome of future referenda we do know that this issue is not going to go away. This essay is an attempt to articulate the issues and concerns that continue to give rise to proposals to legalize physician-assisted suicide and euthanasia.

ANALYZING THE PROPOSALS

Ethical analysis of proposals like Proposition 161 generally begins by recalling the long accepted prohibition against killing. To date, people attacking proposals such as 161 use three arguments. First, arguing from either religious or humanistic bases, opponents of legalized "aid in dying" seek to demonstrate that there is something about the nature of the human (e.g., that human authority is limited) and of human life (e.g., its sanctity or inherent dignity) that precludes both the intention to kill and actions taken to realize that intention. Second, opponents of these kinds of proposals rail at those who seek to expand the boundaries of personal autonomy in an attempt to "preserve

184

dignity." Third, a great deal of attention is devoted to convincing people that, because of the potential that exists for abuse of nonautonomous, vulnerable persons, proposals like 161 should not be approved. What we fail to recognize, however, is that the expressed concerns about self-determination and freedom from pain resulting in propositions like 161 are only symptoms of a much more significant problem. There are deeply rooted and sensitive concerns that lead people to the conclusion that the only way to preserve dignity in the face of long-term, debilitating, terminal illness is to request and receive "aid in dying." As long as these more basic issues are not dealt with effectively and compassionately, proposals like Proposition 161 will continue to make their way to state and national ballots.

IDENTIFYING THE DEEPER ISSUES

Ernest Becker noted in his Pulitzer Prize winning book, *The Denial of Death*, that "the idea of death, the fear of it, haunts the human animal like nothing else; it is a mainspring of human activity—activity designed largely to avoid the fatality of death, to overcome it by denying in some way that it is the final destiny for man."[2] It is not only biological death that we fear. As a society, we seem to dread most forms of diminishment. Our attitudes toward the normal process of aging as well as toward increasing debility and disability bespeak this anxiety. Moreover, the pervasive conviction that productivity is the measure of both personal and social worth often gives rise to the conclusion that human dignity is somehow dependent on one's usefulness, particularly in economic terms. When the ability to produce or contribute actively wanes and dependency increases, for whatever reason, we often conclude that human dignity thereby is diminished or extinguished altogether. Perhaps the noted lack of social commitment to provide appropriate care for the aging, the terminally ill, and the dying is a reflection of this underlying inability to accept diminishment and death as natural parts of life.

Working within this broad societal framework are health care professionals who come to the professions embodying many of these same fears and anxieties about human diminishment and death. As a result, the way health care services are provided often reflects this fear. For example, most health care services, whether in acute care or long-term care facilities, are provided according to the paradigm of the "medical model" of illness. Accordingly, illness is viewed as a foreign invader to be overcome by the use of medical technology with the goal of returning the person to his or her former self. While this model may be appropriate when dealing with acute illness, it is inappropriate when applied to chronic, debilitating, or terminal illness. In fact, it can be quite harmful for it fails to recognize that the person's identity is constituted through the experience of chronic or debilitating illness. Unlike the person who is returned to her former state of well-being, and therefore her former self, following the removal of a diseased organ, the person with Lou Gehrig's or Alzheimer's disease *becomes who he is and will be* as he experiences and deals with the disease on an ongoing basis. Thus, persons with chronic, long-term, debilitating illness can be harmed gravely by physicians and other health care professionals who fail to accept that all illness is not remediable.

In addition, the failure on the part of many in medicine to recognize and apply sound ethical criteria for the use and nonuse of life-sustaining interventions often leads to a technologic assault on irreversible illness. And at the same time that many persons are forced to go through a protracted dying process because of medicine's unwillingness to "let go," there is often also a reluctance to ensure that the person's dying is as comfortable as possible. Basing the cautious and often ineffective use of pain control measures on the fear of "hastening death" or of "causing addiction," some physicians and nurses make the understandably difficult experience of terminal illness something to be dreaded and, if possible, avoided. For many individuals, then, the prospect of debilitating, long-term, or terminal illness is an understandably frightening one. Many persons fear becoming a "burden" to others. Few people fail to recognize that long-term illness and the care that it requires can easily bankrupt a family and jeopardize its economic future. Moreover, there is the constant fear of becoming a nonproductive, noncontributing member of family or community. The "warehousing" of persons that often occurs in long-term care settings contributes to this apprehension.

The most pervasive fear is that of becoming a "captive" of a system that is often ill-equipped or unwilling to provide appropriate, compassionate care at life's end. Reflecting on the recent experiences of Nancy Beth Cruzan and Christine Busalacchi, many people conclude that the only way to overcome the mindless application of health care technology at life's end is to ensure release from the system by requiring medically-assisted killing.

Finally, the potential for loss of control looms large in the minds of many when they contemplate long-term and terminal illness. This seems to be particularly true of younger persons facing such illness. As long-term or terminal illness progresses, persons often must relinquish much of the control they once enjoyed over even the most basic of human functions. As a result, they are forced to turn to concerned and caring others to do for them what they can no longer do for themselves. But in many cases there are no "caring others" willing or available to provide such care. The lack of community and the isolation experienced by many today frequently means that when persons are most in need they often are surrounded only by strangers. When this is the case, the sense of loss of control is magnified. The request to be killed then becomes an attempt to reclaim some degree of power, and thereby dignity, in the midst of powerlessness.

CONCLUSION

While initiatives like Proposition 161 may be defeated for the present, others will be proposed in the future. But legalizing assisted suicide and euthanasia is not the way to address the concerns and fears of persons who face the prospects of long term, debilitating, and terminal illness. Rather, we must realize that diminishment, dying, and death are natural parts of human life. When the limits to the ability to overcome such realities have been met, then persons should be helped to live well even while dying. This requires several things. First, we must recognize that the dignity of the human person is inalienable and cannot be diminished by any form of illness or disability. The tragedy is that too frequently persons with debilitating or terminal illness are treated without regard for their dignity. We must correct this. Second, life-sustaining interventions should be used in a reasonable and prudent manner. The inability to heal or cure in all instances should not be interpreted by health care professionals as failure. Rather, caring for debilitated or dying persons should be seen as an opportunity to offer compassionate presence to the person who enters the transformative process of dying and death. Providing adequate control of pain and discomfort, as well as offering a community of care and support willing to accompany the terminally ill and dying person through the experience are the ethically appropriate responses to these human realities. Only when all persons can expect to receive such care if faced with long-term, debilitating, and terminal illness will we silence the voices calling for legalized killing.

NOTES

1. The California Death With Dignity Act. Amendment to the California Civil Code, Title 10.5, August, 1991.
2. Ernest Backer, *The Denial of Death* (New York: *The Free Press*, 1973), *ix*.

55: Research on Human Embryos: Ethical Perspective

Research upon human embryos is a reality. Is it an ethical practice? Recently four different study groups have evaluated the practice. Analysis of these studies is informative in regard to contemporary ethical methodologies. The scientific study groups publishing reports are: a) Committee of Inquiry into Human Fertilization and Embryology (The Warnock Committee) in the United Kingdom, 1984; b) The Senate Select Committee on The Human Embryo Experimentation Bill, Australia, 1985; c) The Bioethics Summit Conference representing seven member countries of the Economic Summit Conference, 1987; d) A study prepared by the Ministry of Justice in West Germany, 1988.

PRINCIPLES

The human embryo results from penetration of a mature ovum by a sperm, the chromosomes from male and female combining to form a new and unique genetic identity. Though it is possible to conduct research upon the embryo in any stage of development, the stage of development under discussion by the scientific study groups is the first fourteen days of existence. Thus, the study groups were concerned with research upon embryos that are generated in vitro, and never introduced into a womb. At present, embryos generated in this manner may be sustained outside the womb for about ten to twelve days. However, we can envision this time being extended indefinitely through the proper technology. The source of embryos for research, for the most part, would be "extra" embryos resulting from fertilization of multiple ova resulting from in-vitro fertilization. However, the fertilization of ova with the express intent of using the developing embryo for research purposes is not unknown and is approved by at least one study group.

The study groups found the distinction between therapeutic and nontherapeutic research most significant. If this distinction is applied to research involving human embryos, a *therapeutic research* on an embryo is carried out with the aim or object of acting in the best interests of the embryo that is the subject of the procedure (for example, correcting genetic defects).

Nontherapeutic experimentation does not directly benefit the individual embryo undergoing the procedure. Knowledge gained from the research may ultimately benefit future embryos by advancing the understanding of human generation or by improving medical therapy. Witnesses appearing before the study committees agreed that nontherapeutic experimentation on an embryo, at least for the present, is intrusive and destructive of that embryo.

DISCUSSION

There was no disagreement among the study groups in regard to therapeutic research. If the human and social future of the embryo is respected and curative or diagnostic results are intended, the research would be acceptable. At present, there does not seem to be any therapeutic research projects designed for embryos that will never be introduced into a womb.

In regard to nontherapeutic research, however, there was great disagreement. The Australian study group declared: "The Committee concludes that the respect due to the embryo from the process of fertilization onwards requires its protection from destructive nontherapeutic experimentation." In Germany, the Ministry of Justice reached a like conclusion recommending legislation that would make it a criminal offense to engage in any research that could be considered harmful to a human embryo.

The United Kingdom study group recommended that nontherapeutic research be permitted up to fourteen days from fertilization. The international committee recognized the "preciousness of the human embryo," but allowed nontherapeutic research if it were "regulated by appropriate guidelines administered by a competent authority."

Why the difference of ethical evaluation for nontherapeutic research upon human embryos? The difference does not rest in a radical disagreement over the nature of the human embryo, all groups accepting it as a separate living entity with genetic human identity. Nor is there disagreement in regard to the value of the knowledge that might be gained from this type of research. There is severe disagreement, however, in regard to protecting the human embryo from harm and destruction. What rights of the embryo must be respected in face of the rights of the human community to scientific knowledge? In discussing this conflict of rights, some groups use a utilitarian approach, emphasizing the good to be attained, rather than the good of the subject involved in the research. In this system the goal of ethical deliberation is to "balance rights": no inalienable rights of the embryo being recognized. This history of utilitarianism indicates that it minimizes human worth and the value of the individual. Using this system of ethical evaluation, Dame Mary Warnock declared: "In a calculation of harms and benefits the very early embryo need not be counted."[1]

Opposed to this method of ethical evaluation are systems that consider the human being worthy of respect and protection, even if knowledge or other goods must be sacrificed. According to this method of ethical evaluation some goods or rights are considered so basic and significant that they cannot be balanced with other rights nor be sacrificed for other goods. *The Helsinki*

Statement of the World Health Organization, in regard to the ethics of research, summed up this ethical approach when it declared: "Concern for the interests of the subject must always prevail over the interest of science and society."[2]

The ethical theory that places the good of the patient or subject before the good of science or society is part of the heritage of medicine. When have you heard a physician or scientist whom you admire declare: "I don't care what happens to my patients or subjects, as long as we get some useful information."

CONCLUSION

Everything that is possible is not necessarily beneficial. When assessing benefit, we must be careful to respect the inalienable rights of individuals and not merely balance these rights with other goods.

NOTES

1. Report of the Committee of Inquiry into Human Fertilization and Embryology. HMSO, London, 7/18/84.

2. Declaration of Helsinki, World Medical Association, 1964 and 1975, *Encyclopedia of Bioethics* (4), 1769.

56: The Oregon Health Care Plan: Some Questions

In the state of Oregon recently, a seven-year-old boy died of leukemia. Shortly before his death, state health officials refused public funds for a potentially life-prolonging bone marrow transplant. In the same state, a young mother was refused public funding for a liver transplant. Both actions resulted from a new policy of state health officials to refuse funding for bone marrow, pancreas, heart or liver transplants. The decisions in Oregon have been portrayed as a preview of the decisions that will soon be necessary by officials in other states and by officials representing the federal government. The economic decisions that limit the access to health care have ethical implications. People will live or die as a result of these decisions. With this in mind, a closer investigation of the decisions in Oregon are in order.

PRINCIPLES

Is there a general principle that will ensure an ethical distribution of public funds to those in need of health care? In Oregon, the painful decisions to withhold funds was based upon the assumption that basic health care should be provided before advanced or experimental care. Hence, the state officials in Oregon pointed out that basic health care was being provided for 24,000 more low income people without any increase of funds by reason of the new policy. Moreover, they pointed out, "1500 pregnant women will receive prenatal care with the same amount of money that would pay for thirty organ transplants." Many commentators and editorial writers, applauding the wisdom and courage of the Oregon allotment policy, declared that Oregon should be a model for federal agencies faced with the same decisions. A consensus seems to be present in the public forum then, that basic care for the most people possible should be the principle upon which access to health care for lower income people is determined.

The Oregon decisions occur at a time when many people are searching for principles to regulate the amount of our national assets devoted to health care. In his provocative book, *Setting Limits*, Daniel Callahan maintains that a new norm for funding health care for the aging must be developed. At present, the health care research and therapy in the United States seems to be directed toward keeping people alive as long as possible, no matter what degree of function they might retain. Callahan persuasively questions whether this is a realistic norm, given the limited resources of our society and the certainty of death. He suggests that a more valid norm would be to afford as many people as possible the opportunity to live a beneficial life. Making such a radical readjustment in health care planning would direct funds away from the aging toward the younger members of society. Callahan realizes that his idea is prophetic, stating that it will not be accepted until his grandchildren are adults.

DISCUSSION

The policies initiated in Oregon give some guidance for the future. Moreover, Callahan's ideas, which are explained much more intelligently and compassionately in his book, must be considered as the issue of allotting funds for research and health care therapy is discussed. However, both in Oregon and in Callahan's discussion, there is a vital question that has not been considered sufficiently. At the present time, are we devoting a fair share of national assets to health care for low income people? While we may posit limited resources for health care, have we reached the reasonable limits of our resources? For the past fifteen years, the proportion of our gross national product (GNP) devoted to health care has been a prominent discussion topic. This is a significant percentage of the GNP to items that can only be deemed ephermal. Are there many goods included in the GNP that are more important than access to health care? Moreover, it is that simple to distinguish between basic and advanced health care? If the criterion for distinguishing between basic and advanced health care is the success of the procedure, then some types of organ transplant may at present be designated as basic care and other types will soon be in that category.

A prominent health care economist, Uwe Reinhardt, when testifying before the Senate Commission on Aging, pointed out that Americans are delighted when figures indicate that the automobile industry is flourishing because this "is good for the economy and good for the country." He asks whether the same attitude is not fitting insofar as health care is concerned. While not fostering a *laissez faire* attitude toward health care costs, we must admit Reinhardt is right in one regard. If we compare present and past percentages of the GNP devoted to health care, we are comparing apples and oranges. Though medicine still has the same goals it had forty years ago, the means and methods of reaching these goals have changed significantly.

CONCLUSION

According to the great Swiss theologian Karl Barth, a society must be judged upon its willingness to care for its weak and impoverished members. Although health care procedures should be carefully evaluated for cost efficiency, and although the function of a patient should be considered when evaluating the effectiveness of health care procedures, it seems equally important to evaluate whether or not our states and the federal government are at present devoting enough of our assets to offering access to health care for lower income people.

57: The Oregon Plan: Portents for the Future?

After much deliberation, the Bush Administration rejected the Oregon Plan, an innovative proposal to revise the Medicaid Program in the state of Oregon.[1] The Plan proposes to increase the number of people covered by Medicaid by limiting the medical and surgical procedures available to Medicaid patients. Thus patients eligible for Medicaid insurance would receive basic care, but advanced care, such as organ transplants would not be available. As the first step in defining "basic" health care, 709 common medical and surgical procedures were evaluated according to their projected benefits and cost. Second, the state legislature allocated funds to cover the procedures that were considered to be basic. In the original plan, procedures 1–587 were covered, but that number could be reduced or expanded in the future depending upon the funds allocated. Procedures unavailable to Medicaid patients would often be available to those with private insurance.

The Plan also proposes to increase the number of people and families covered under private health insurance by requiring all businesses to offer health insurance to their employees. The aforementioned system of evaluating medical and surgical procedures would in time be applied to those in private insurance programs and in Medicare. Of course, those in private insurance programs could contract for more extensive coverage, if they or their employers paid extra premiums. At first glance, the Oregon Plan seems to solve some of the more pressing problems involved in providing adequate access to health care in the United States. It increases the number of people covered by Medicaid, and it defines a "basic" set of health care procedures that should be available to all. However, officials of the Department of Health and Human Services (HHS) rejected the Oregon Plan. This essay will explain briefly why the Oregon Plan was rejected by the federal government, and then point out some lessons that the formulation and rejection of this plan offer for the future.

PRINCIPLES

The Oregon Plan would have reduced the medical benefits that each state is required to provide for poor pregnant women and their children. Sara Rosenbaum points out that the United States Congress has mandated that states that participate in the Medicaid program *must* provide all necessary health care for persons receiving payments under the Aid to Families with Dependent

194

Children Program (AFDC), virtually all of whom are women and children.[2] Participating states must also provide all health care required for aged, blind, and disabled recipients of Supplemental Security Income (SSI). In addition, laws enacted in recent years mandate health care for all pregnant women, infants, children under age six with family incomes below 133% of the federal poverty level, as well as for children ages six to nineteen with family incomes below 100% of the federal poverty level. As a result of the amendments to the original Medicaid legislation, the states' authority to cover less than all medically necessary health services for certain groups of people has been eliminated.

When refusing to approve the Oregon Plan for the aforementioned reasons, Secretary Louis Sullivan of HHS stated that the plan would discriminate against disabled people. Because "quality of life" is part of the rating evaluation formula, he maintained that the Plan would be contrary to the Americans with Disabilities Act, which requires that medical treatment must not be withheld solely because of present or predictable disabilities. Citing the list of medical procedures, he declared that "babies weighing more than 500 grams would be eligible for extensive life support while babies weighing less than 500 grams would not receive treatment because of their predicted 'quality of life' if they survived." Other people wishing to reject the Plan cited the discrimination that would result in the care of babies born with eminently treatable disabilities such as spina bifida. Babies covered by private insurance would receive treatment while those covered only by Medicaid might not receive treatment because the procedure might not be considered "basic care," due to reduced funding by the Oregon legislature.

DISCUSSION

Though it seems to contradict some of the recent federal laws, the Oregon Plan has focused national attention on important problems that confront the people of the United States as we seek to reform the provision of health care.

1. First and foremost, the Plan reveals dramatically some of the shortcomings of the present "system" of health care in the United States. Even if the Plan were given a waiver from federal law there would still be many problems in providing adequate access to health care for all citizens of Oregon. Location of health care professionals and health care facilities have a telling effect upon the provision of adequate access to health care. No mention is made in the Plan of these structural needs. An even more important problem revealed by the Plan is the method of funding health care. The Plan helps us realize that adequate access will not be achieved by "robbing Peter to pay Paul." Will sufficient funds be available if waste is eliminated and health care

costs reduced? Perhaps, but the Plan doesn't address the issues of waste and medical care inflation. A comprehensive health care program must devote more thought to incorporating the market factors that are the most effective way of controlling costs. The Oregon Plan seems to assume that the present method of funding health care is sound and that all it needs is touching up at the edges. For example, there is no consideration of a "single party payor," which would eliminate some of the administrative costs for health care. In sum, the Plan seems to prolong the assumption that private health insurance, financed by employer and administrated by private health insurance companies, is an essential and beneficial element of health care. These assumptions must be questioned if a true renewal in health care is to be developed.

2. The Plan shows the difficulty of defining "basic health care procedures." Almost every one of the many plans to renew U.S. health care state that "basic health care should be provided for all." But none of the other plans have sought to define and describe the meaning of the term "basic care." The Oregon Plan seeks to do so and in the process demonstrates that determining the procedures that constitute "basic health care" is a complex process. Not only the cost of the procedure must be considered but also the extent and duration of the benefit, given the condition of the patient. Moreover, a better understanding of the role "quality of life" plays in determining basic health care must be developed. Secretary Sullivan's point concerning extensive life support for babies above and below 500 grams is well taken. On the other hand, does it make sense to offer extensive life support to any baby weighing less than 500 grams? Declaring that basic health care can be defined implies that definite financial limits must be set for national health care expenditures. To date, the U.S. health care system has been conducted as though unlimited funds are available, at least for those with private or public insurance. Devoting an excessive portion of the Gross National Product to health care makes it impossible to devote adequate funds to other significant needs, such as education, housing, improvement of the environment, and replacement of the "infrastructure."

3. The Plan demonstrates the anguish caused by explicit rationing of health care. At present, health care in the United States is rationed implicitly, the system being unable to care for people without insurance. About 15% of our population, that is about 35–40 million people, do not have adequate access to health care. As a result, they experience ill health more often than the rest of the population, making it more difficult for them to work, go to school, and lead fulfilling lives, than it is for the rest of the population. Moreover, people without adequate access to health care die at earlier ages from diseases and illnesses

that could be controlled or even healed were health care provided. Through explicit rationing of health care, decisions will be made that will shorten the life of some people now receiving adequate access to care. The problem called to the forefront by explicit rationing was expressed eloquently by a friend of mine: "Rationing health care for older, debilitated people approaching death is a worthwhile idea, but leave my Mom out of it!"

CONCLUSION

An overwhelming number of people in the United States agree that the provision of health care needs *radical* change. Though it is innovative, the Oregon Plan is not radical enough. Insofar as many issues in health care are concerned, such as financing and delivery of health care, the Oregon Plan seems to endorse the status quo. But the Plan does illustrate that radical renewal of our health care system might be considered as the thirteenth labor of Hercules.

NOTES

1. The Clinton Administration approved experimentation with the Oregon Plan. However, because of financial limitations and a change in the makeup of the Oregon legislature, implementation of the plan has languished.
2. Sara Rosenbaum, "Mothers and Children Last: The Oregon Medicaid Experiment," *American Journal of Law and Medicine* XVII: 1 & 2 (1992), 97–126.

58: IVF and Surrogate Motherhood: Methods of Ethical Evaluation

Recently in Aberdeen, South Dakota, Arlette Schweitzer, 42 years old, gave birth to twins. Not an unusual event, save for one factor. The twins were the result of in vitro fertilization (IVF) and embryo transplant, using ova from her daughter, Christa, and sperm from her son-in-law, Kevin Uchytil. In other words, through the assistance of technicians and technology, Arlette Schweitzer became the "mother" of her genetic grandchildren. While a woman in South Africa played the same role in the generation of triplets in 1987, the case was the first of its kind in the United States. Once again, this process of fertilization, gestation, and birth prompted an evaluation of in vitro fertilization and surrogate "motherhood" in general, and the Schweitzer-Uchytil collaboration in particular. In this essay, we shall recount some of the discussion and seek to contribute to the discussion from an ethical perspective. As well as presenting a unique family situation, the case offers a fascinating example of the way in which different ethical methods are utilized in the United States and the varying results of these different methods.

PRINCIPLES

Most people commenting upon the Schweitzer-Uchytil collaboration focused exclusively upon the ultimate intentions of the person involved. This is a most popular form of ethical evaluation in the United States. If the facts and the outcome of the Schweitzer-Uchytil case are evaluated from a the viewpoint of intention, then the action would be "good." Two young married persons wish to have a child, but because the mother was born without a uterus they are unable to generate children through the natural process of sexual intercourse. By means of IVF and transplant of the zygote into the womb of Christa's mother, they are able to use their own genetic material to cooperate in the production of new persons. Arlette Schweitzer stated that carrying the babies "was an act of love, I never had any second thoughts." Hence the ultimate intentions of all parties seems to be above reproach.

The problem with evaluating human actions solely from the viewpoint of the ultimate intention is that almost any action or group of actions joined together by an ultimate intention might be evaluated as "good" if the intention is good. One vivid memory of mine from the Fifties recalls an academic type defending the actions of Adolph Hitler because the ultimate intention of all his actions was "the good of the Fatherland." Without questioning the ultimate intentions of the people involved in the Schweitzer-Uchytil case, it seems a more thorough ethical analysis is needed. The impact upon the overall well-being of all persons involved in the series of actions that produced the desired effect should be analyzed. The term "overall well-being" implies that we must evaluate the impact of the free human acts upon the functions or capacities of the persons involved; that is, the physical, psychological, social, and creative (spiritual) capacities of the persons.

Probing the impact of actions upon the physical, psychological, social, and creative functions or capacities of the person is not always easy. Because these human functions or capacities exist in the unity of a person, the impact upon the capacities or functions of the person should not be analyzed disjunctively, but rather in an integrated manner. To put it another way, the aforementioned functions of the human personality are related as dimensions of a cube, not as layers in a cake. While a layer of cake may be removed and the remains would still be a cake, if a dimension of a cube is removed the cube ceases to be. Though one function may be more important than another, for example, the creative function is considered the most important because to some extent it is directive of the others, no function can be sacrificed for another. Could we think and love (creative functions) without our bodies? Our physiological function, though in some ways the least "dignified" level of human function, must not be manipulated or sacrificed unless for the good of the whole body. For this reason, to save the whole body, we consider the removal of diseased organs a good action. But we do not approve of mutilating our bodies for money (social good). For this reason we consider selling the organs of a living person, such as a kidney, as unethical. We are not persons (spirits) merely existing in bodies, rather we are person because we have bodies. As persons we are an integrated unity of body and spirit.

DISCUSSION

Does this method of ethical evaluation help us in evaluating the case in question? The principal persons involved in IVF using genetic material supplied by a married couple, later completed by embryo transplant, are the wife and husband, the woman who serves as surrogate, and the children resulting if the process is successful. Briefly, let us consider the impact upon these people.

The husband and wife who supply the genetic material for the new children may impose unforeseen burdens upon themselves. Paul Lauritzen, speaking for himself and his wife, sums up the experience of their efforts to generate children through technological processes by saying: "The process of reproduction in a clinical environment (causes) a way of thinking of ourselves and our world in terms that are incompatible with intimacy . . . once procreation is separated from sexual intercourse, it is difficult not to treat the process of procreation as the production of an object to which one has the right as a producer. It is also difficult under these circumstances to place the end above the means: effectiveness in accomplishing one's goal can easily become the sole criterion by which decisions are made." ("What Price Parenthood," *Hastings Center Report*), March/April 1990).[1]

As nature (evolution) has designed the act of generation (sexual intercourse) as a fully human act, it involves all the functions of the persons who come together to perform the action. Moreover, it requires and enhances intimacy between the two people. As a result of intimacy, the couple willingly gestate, nurture, and educate the embryo, infant, child. If intimacy is lacking as the Lauritzens avow, will generation through IVF and surrogate gestation be beneficial for parents and child? The objection to IVF may be phrased in this way: Will the IVF method result in the deprivation of some vital familial goods that loving intercourse will provide? When IVF is used in the process of fertilization of genetic material, if a child results, the child is not generated in a human fashion; rather it is manufactured. Will this make a difference? Is it possible to inflict harm upon ourselves and others by circumventing or ignoring the process of nature. By ignoring nature, we have seen the damage we have done to our environment. Are we setting ourselves up for the same type of disaster by ignoring the ecology of human generation? Finally, as another drawback of assisted reproduction Lauritzen maintains: "The cycle of hope and then despair that repeats itself in unsuccessful fertility treatments can become unbearable."

In regard to the gestational mother who is to nurture the infants for nine months and then give them up, it seems a serious psychological, social, and creative burden also may be imposed upon her. As indicated in the famous Baby M case a few years ago, surrogate motherhood demands that the woman who is the gestational mother not act like a mother. The bonding that occurs between a mother and infant in the womb is stronger and more long lasting than any other human bond. Is it beneficial or even possible for a woman to act like a mother for nine months, and then severe the deepest human ties and pretend she is not the mother of her child for the rest of her life? The children of IVF and surrogate transplant may also be deprived in the process. A sense of identity needed for healthy personal development is founded upon the knowledge that one knows one's parents. The development of identity in each person results from gestation, nurturing, and education. These three elements are a continuum. Will separating the elements of this process injure children? Will IVF and gestational surrogacy weaken family bonds as children grow older and wonder about their "real" parents?

CONCLUSION

Coping with infertility is a difficult burden for married people. Clearly, some methods of coping with this burden will be more beneficial than others. Coping through IVF and embryo transplant to a surrogate mother may not be as problem-free a method of coping as once believed.

NOTE

1. Paul Lauritzen, "What Price Parenthood," *Hastings Center Report*, March/ April 1990, vol. 20, p. 38ff.

59: Conceiving One Child to Save Another

Abe and Mary Ayala, a California couple in their mid-forties, did not plan to have another child. But they changed their minds when their seventeen-year old daughter, Anissa, was diagnosed as having leukemia, a cancer of the blood cells that can sometimes be cured by transplanting bone marrow cells from a compatible donor. Because the medical team could not find a suitable donor among relatives or friends, the Ayalas decided to have another child, taking a one in four chance that the newborn child would be a compatible bone marrow donor for Anissa. The one in four gamble seems to be paying off. Prenatal testing indicates that the female fetus will be a compatible bone marrow donor.

When the Ayala story became public, medical ethicists were consulted and some criticized the venture because the newly conceived child was being treated as a "means," not as an "end." In response to the observations of the ethicists, several media persons affirmed the right of the Ayalas to do whatever they desired as long as love is their motive. At the same time, some columnists berated the ethicists for offering opinions from an ivory tower. Can we evaluate the actions of the Ayalas from an ethical perspective? Does ethics have anything to offer in regard to such a personal and emotion-laden decision?

PRINCIPLES

Though there is no method of ethical evaluation that eliminates emotional reactions, there are distinctions and considerations that may help to minimize them. First of all, it is necessary to distinguish the remote intention or purpose of the act in question from the intention or purpose embodied in the act itself. If only the remote intention of an action is emphasized to the exclusion of the proximate intention expressed in the act itself, then one can justify just about anything. If I rob poor widows to pay for my college education and consider only the remote intention, then robbing widows might be put forth as a good action because it enabled me to obtain a college education. Discussions concerning the morality of abortion often break down because of failure to make this distinction. In the case of the Ayalas, their desire to prolong the life of Anissa is a good intention. But the means they utilize to prolong her life must be evaluated in their own right. Is it ethically acceptable to conceive

202

a child mainly with the intention of providing therapy for another child? This is the ethical issue under consideration.

When assessing an action with emotional overtones, it is helpful to step back and say: "What if everybody performed the action with the same purpose in mind?" Emmanuel Kant recommended that a similar question be asked when forming ethical norms. What if every child were conceived as a means to prolong the life of other living persons? What would this do to our society and to the self-esteem of children as they progress to maturity?

Another approach that helps to evaluate an emotion-laden action is to consider the action from a perspective that all would consider acceptable. Then consider the action in question from a perspective that all would consider perverse. Finally, compare the action in question to both good and perverse actions to determine whether it more closely resembles the good action or the perverse action. For example, it seems that if a child is conceived as a sign and result of the mutual love of the parents and is nurtured and educated with the intention of helping the child attain human fulfillment, then most would agree that this is a good action. However, all would agree that conceiving children in order to sell them into slavery would be wrong; wrong because it debases and devalues the worth and dignity of the human persons who will be slaves. Even if the parents plead poverty and state that their children will have a more comfortable life in slavery than if they had stayed with their poor parents, the act of generating human beings with the intention of selling them into slavery is simply unacceptable. A child should never be considered the property of the parents. Clearly, generating a child as a potential bone marrow donor is not exactly the same as conceiving a child in order to sell him into slavery. But does the intention of the Ayalas resemble more closely the good or the perverse intention mentioned above?

DISCUSSION

Mrs. Ayala responded to remarks of ethicists by saying: "We are going to love our baby. Our baby is going to have more love than she probably can put up with." While there is no desire to question the overall dispositions of the Ayalas', the aforementioned statement illustrates the difficulty of using accurately the word "love" in the English language. In English, we convey three different human actions through the one word "love." In Greek, three words are used to convey these three types of love: *philia*, *eros*, and *agape*. The significance of this examination of words and concepts is that the deepest form of human love, *agape*, is the type of love we predicate between parents and children. *Agape* is incompatible with self-serving intentions. Can we say we have the deepest form of love for another (*agape*) if we are going to use that other person to achieve goals that we have determined without consulting the person in question? Thus, the need for more accurate distinctions and soul searching evaluation when we use the word "love" to justify human actions.

Stepping back from the immediate question once more, let us consider the activity and outlook of the physicians who advised the Ayalas. While they remained behind the scenes insofar as the news stories were concerned, we surmise that they were deeply involved in the decisions to create a "suitable" bone marrow donor. Once again, we face the question: Is the goal of medicine to prolong life as long as possible, no matter what means are used? Or is the goal of medicine to help people pursue a better life, the worth and dignity of all persons being respected in the process? If one opts for prolonging life as the ultimate purpose of medical care, then the patient (and/or family) is often subjected to therapy with no view to the values and priorities of the person. Most cases of overtreatment as death approaches are examples of the "prolonging life at all costs" outlook. In the immediate future, as the ability to prolong life increases, for example, through mechanical devices such as the artificial heart, or through xenografts, the question of human benefit must be put in the forefront of medical and ethical decisions. What risks and burdens are to be endured to prolong one's own life or the life of another?

CONCLUSION

Finally, do ethicists have any role in commenting upon personal and emotion-laden decisions that have ethical ramifications? Seemingly, they have as much right to comment as do newspaper columnists, but saying this doesn't answer the question. Clearly, the observations of ethicists are offered more effectively before than after the fact. If offered after the fact, the observations must be thorough and circumspect or they will be lost in the emotional reaction to which they give rise.

60: Use of Fetal Tissue in Research and Therapy

The ethical assessment of using fetal tissue for research/therapeutic purposes is, at first glance, deceptively easy. Regardless of the source of the tissue, the potential good to be done would seem to require that otherwise "wasted" fetal remains be put to some good use, whether that be for pure research or for the treatment of identified persons suffering from conditions such as Parkinson's disease, Alzheimer's disease, brain damage, or spinal cord injuries. The fact that some tissue might come from electively aborted fetuses can appear to be of little consequence in light of the hoped for good to be achieved. And indeed, if one relies primarily on a utilitarian approach (i.e., an approach that argues that the good you are seeking to accomplish can be pursued *even if* the means to that good are evil) then one can appear to justify use of fetal tissue from any available source.

However, traditional medical ethics has relied on principles other than utility in determining what is/is not ethically appropriate in the practice of medicine in both the research and therapeutic settings. Thus, principles such as nonmaleficence and beneficence require that physicians refrain from harming persons; that they do not choose to do evil even if some good can be produced in the process; and that they always act in the best interests of persons.

In applying these principles to the ethical assessment of the use of fetal tissue in research and therapy, it is necessary to address the source of the tissue. Once the source has been identified, then the question to be answered is: "Is use of tissue from this source ethically justified?"

Generally, tissue for such purposes is available from either spontaneously aborted or electively aborted fetuses. In cases where spontaneous abortion is the source, it would seem that one would be ethically justified in using the tissue for either research or therapeutic purposes providing, of course, that suitable respect is shown to the fetal remains and that appropriate consent is obtained from the parents.

The ethical evaluation of using tissue from elective/induced abortions is made recognizing that such abortion constitutes an evil in itself. This recognition requires that a number of questions be asked in making the ethical assessment. Does the use of electively aborted fetal tissue support the evil of abortion? Does use of this tissue constitute complicity in the evil of abortion? Does the use of this tissue further the growth of the abortion industry to the extent that such use should be ethically proscribed?

Because of the potential for good from use of this tissue, I would like to answer "no" to such questions—such use does not constitute ethically unacceptable cooperation in abortion. But caution must be exercised here to ensure that the evil of abortion does not become institutionalized in our society because of an implicit justification that it gains as we attempt to rationalize the use of electively aborted fetal tissue in the pursuit of some good(s).

Such a cautious approach must take account of the following. First, without the availability of fetal tissue there would be no possibility of benefit. Thus, any separation between research/therapeutic goals and abortion created by legal or other means is simply a fiction. Second, even if initially only fetal tissue from ethically acceptable sources is used, once the therapeutic possibilities become evident, the need and demand for wider availability of tissue will grow exponentially beyond what can be provided from spontaneous abortions.

Third, the often painful decision to have an abortion could be mitigated by knowledge that some good could come from such a choice. The possibility of such relief could in turn lessen the reluctance to choose death over life when women are faced with such options.

Recall the recent arguments made in favor of using anencephalic infants as organ donors—arguments made in favor of expanding the criteria for determining death in these newborns so that their organs would be more useful for others. The rationale for this approach (at least in part) was that the parents could feel that their baby's life or death had some meaning. But what was understood as the source of that meaning? The baby's usefulness to another in need of a transplant.

Since medicine and its developing technologies are oriented to benefiting persons, the temptation will always exist to assess the appropriateness of methods for providing that benefit purely according to a utilitarian calculus, which always includes the ability to use evil as a means to achieve a good. Such an approach, however, threatens to supplant the fundamental ethical norms that inform traditional medical ethics (i.e., do not harm and benefit when able). Furthermore, utilitarian thinking tries to convince us that we may be justified in setting aside our commonly held views of what is morally appropriate given a potential benefit of great enough significance. And that is the real danger here.

Unless great caution is exercised, we risk initiating a self-perpetuating process of justification whereby two things occur, both of which are equally unacceptable.

First, the "evil" (i.e., individual abortions or the abortion industry in general) that we do/participate in, in the pursuit of the good (research/therapy) looses its significance for us "as evil" . . . or at least it takes on the identity of one of those "necessary evils" that we no longer find troubling.

Second, the many "lesser" concerns (e.g., paying for fetal tissue to increase the supply thereby increasing the number of abortions or providing incentives for delaying abortion until the second or third trimesters in order to have more developed, more useful tissue/organs) become nonconcerns in light of the good that we propose to do.

The separation between the good that is hoped for and the evil used as a means to achieve that good must be complete and substantial. Until it is, the ethical appropriateness of using fetal tissue obtained from elective abortions (and perhaps even spontaneous abortions) will remain questionable.

61: New Therapies for Ectopic Pregnancy

Historically, the ethical evaluation of the treatment of ectopic pregnancy has been made by application of the principle of double effect. Removal of the involved fallopian tube by salpingectomy was allowed, even though the tube contained a previable embryo, because it was argued that the direct aim and intention of the surgeon was the removal of the diseased tube and reversal of the condition that threatened the life of the woman. The subsequent embryo death was described as "indirect" because while it could not be avoided, it was neither willed nor "done directly."[1] The fact that, until quite recently, diagnosis of ectopic pregnancy generally was not made until tubal rupture was at least a possibility grounded the claim that a proportionately grave reason existed for removing the affected tube. However, if it was not clear that immediate surgical intervention provided "notably greater probability" of saving the life of the woman,[2] physicians were counseled to wait and watch and allow the embryo to grow.

The direct purpose or immediate effect of the procedure was clearly established by asking, "what is it that the treatment does. . . . what is its aim or purpose?" Whether salpingectomy was performed before or after rupture had occurred, it was argued that the direct purpose/effect of the surgery was to avoid or contain hemorrhage and thus remove serious threat to the life of the mother.

Today, improved diagnostic capabilities allow for detection of ectopic pregnancy often before significant tubal damage has occurred. New conservative surgical and medical techniques such as linear salpingotomy and methotrexate make it *possible* to intervene early in the course of an ectopic pregnancy and correct the pathology often without removing the fallopian tube in hopes of preserving fertility.

PRINCIPLES

These new capabilities raise new ethical questions. Can the death of the embryo that occurs as a result of using the newer treatment modalities continue to be described as "indirect?" Can early intervention that occurs before the life of the mother is *actually* threatened be justified? Can the preservation of fertility constitute a sufficient reason for allowing an intervention that will have as an effect, albeit an indirect effect, the death of the developing embryo?

Three areas of consideration provide the context within which a response to these questions is to be formulated. First, there must be clarity about the basic values that are at stake in situations of ectopic pregnancy. Second, an understanding of the pathology involved and of the way the newer therapies seek to address the pathology is essential. Finally, there should be an appreciation of how the traditional principle of double effect can be applied in current cases of ectopic pregnancy where the circumstances are significantly changed.

DISCUSSION

The primary good at stake in cases of ectopic pregnancy is the good of human life itself, both that of the developing embryo and that of the mother. In the past, since intervention ordinarily was not possible until tubal rupture was threatened or had occurred already, it was clear that the mother's life was in danger from hemorrhage. In addition, even though it was known that early embryonic death was usually the outcome in ectopic pregnancy, it was assumed that a living embryo was contained in the tube and that surgical intervention to save the life of the mother meant unavoidable death for the embryo.

With the advent of more sophisticated diagnostic procedures and the resultant ability to intervene earlier in the course of ectopic pregnancy, the threat to the life of the mother can be significantly reduced. But early diagnosis and treatment does not increase the possibility or probability of preserving the life of the developing embryo. However, these advances do allow for consideration of another value, that of continued fertility, in the overall assessment, both clinical and ethical, or appropriate management of ectopic pregnancy.

The importance of an adequate understanding of the pathology involved in ectopic pregnancy cannot be overstressed in formulating an ethical appraisal of the newer treatment modalities. It is clear that from the moment the fertilized ovum attaches itself to the tubal wall a pathologic condition exists. The outer layer of cells, i.e. the trophoblast, which would normally form the placenta, penetrates the wall of the tube causing erosion of blood vessels. The tube enlarges at the site of initial attachment and as vessels are eroded blood collects and distends the tube making rupture possible.

The newer conservative interventions, both medical and surgical, allow for treatment of *unruptured* tubal pregnancy without destroying the fallopian tube. The aim is to treat the pathologic condition in a way that "preserves as much tubal tissue in a functional state as possible."[3]

The most commonly used conservative surgical intervention is linear salpingotomy. The tube is opened at the site of the unruptured pregnancy and the conceptus is gently detached from the tubal wall and removed.[4] Nonsurgical management can be accomplished by use of a drug such as methotrexate. It acts by inhibiting cellular reproduction and thus is given to prevent further erosion of the tubal wall.[5] The problem, of course, is that even with these improved capabilities we are still dealing with an action that, while seeking to realize a good or value, produces an effect that is evil, i.e. the loss of human life.

In making the ethical assessment, then, the first question to be asked is: What is it that the treatment does. . . . what is its aim or purpose? It seems clear that the interventions, both medical and surgical, aim at correcting the pathology, i.e., destruction of the tubal wall. The therapies propose to limit further tubal damage by removing the invasive tissue or inhibiting its continued growth. The overall intention in using these therapies is that of averting the life-threatening situation that would occur if treatment were not instituted as well as that of protecting, insofar as is possible, the continued fertility of the woman.

Although the action that corrects the pathology, whether surgical or medical, is the same action that brings about the death of the embryo, that death is not the direct effect that is intended. The choice by the physician (and the mother) to use a therapy that increases the possibility of preserving fertility would appear to substantiate this.

CONCLUSION

The use of conservative therapies that allow for early intervention in the course of ectopic pregnancy seems to be ethically justified. This does not mean, of course, that we may exempt ourselves from ongoing analysis and evaluation of developing technology in this area. The time may come when the aberrantly implanted yet still living embryo can be removed and transferred to the uterus where normal growth and development are possible. Such a possibility certainly would change the ethical evaluation of proposed therapies.

NOTES

1. T. Lincoln Bouscaren, S.J., S.T.D. *Ethics of Ectopic Operations* (Milwaukee: The Bruce Publishing Company, 1944).
2. Ibid.
3. Alan H. DeCherney, *Ectopic Pregnancy* (Rockville, MD: Aspen Publishing, Inc., 1986).
4. Ibid., 112.
5. Bruce Sapiro, M.D. "The Nonsurgical Management of Ectopic Pregnancy." Clinical Obstetrics and Gynecology V.30, N.1, March 1987.

62: Cloning (Artificial Twinning): Have We Gone too Far?

On October 26, 1993, the *New York Times* announced that Dr. Jerry Hall and colleagues at George Washington University Medical Center had cloned human embryos. The subsequent firestorm of debate conjured up images of *A Brave New World* and *Jurassic Park*, as well as hundreds of Adolf Hitlers being created from residual hair from his head. However, the technology available today and well into the foreseeable future would not allow for this type of cloning because human cells specialize very early in development. As some *Newsweek* pundits wrote: "A lock of Hitler's hair, even if scientists could extract its DNA, would only give rise to the world's most disgusting hairball."[1] Nevertheless, the artificial creation of twins by means of *in vitro* fertilization techniques in conjunction with cloning methods gives birth to numerous ethical questions.

THE TECHNIQUES AND PURPOSES OF CLONING

The scientists performed their cloning experiments on embryos at various stages of development (up to the 8-cell stage). All of the embryos had genetic malformations because of penetration of the ovum by multiple sperm. Scientists treated these embryos with an enzyme to dissolve the protective shell (the zona pellucida) surrounding the embryonic cells. The identical cells were split apart chemically. The researchers then used sodium alginate to provide a new but artificial zona pellucida which allowed for growth of the newly formed embryos. Some of the cloned embryos reached a maximum of the 32-cell stage of development before they were destroyed as scientists had no intention of implanting the defective embryos.

The main purpose of this type of research is to enhance the possibility of infertile couples to conceive via *in vitro* fertilization. Some infertile couples lack the ability to produce a large number of embryos for implantation. The success rate of implantation for each individual embryo is very low (the overall pregnancy rate is 5–15 percent). Therefore, by increasing the number of embryos implanted through cloning, scientists hope to increase the odds of infertile couples to bear children.

The cloning technology would have other applications. For example, scientists already have the ability to detect genetic defects in embryos at very early cellular development. However, techniques of analysis have an inherent risk of destroying the embryo. Cloning would provide an expendable embryo which could be analyzed and destroyed while safeguarding its twin for implantation. Parents could also freeze cloned embryos and then choose to implant them later after the first child has grown. This leads to the theoretical but unlikely possibility that a woman could give birth to her twin sister some twenty-five years later. Parents could also preserve embryos for later implantation in case the first child dies or needs some type of transplant from an identical donor. This scenario may not be so farfetched since parents in California conceived a child solely for the purpose of providing bone marrow for their teenage daughter suffering from leukemia. In the currently unregulated field of reproductive technologies, one could envision a market for prospective parents who could choose embryos based on what the twin already looks like. And many years in the future, if genetic engineering becomes more refined, one could select for and produce multiple human beings with a particular trait.

THE ETHICAL CONCERNS

The technology of cloning and its application clearly raises many issues about human reproduction, individual identity, and the status of the embryo. Yet the discussion of such issues can be hindered because science and technology are seen as distinct from ethics. Some people believe that science merely involves the pursuit of knowledge. This dissociation of the scientific researcher from ethics fails to recognize that because science impacts on human beings and their values, it must be an ethical endeavor, an endeavor which should not use scientific ends to justify the means, at the expense of human dignity. Hence, in the past, several worldwide ethical commissions from Germany, Australia, and Economic Summit countries have condemned any type of non-therapeutic research on embryos. Once more we must examine critically science's impact on human life, especially that of embryos.

The most significant ethical issue surrounding cloning is the status of the embryo. In the United States where scientists and the public cannot agree on the moral status and rights of the fetus, there certainly will be less respect for the rights of the embryo. As an indication of that, a popular magazine predicted that the new technique of blastomere analysis for genetic defects with subsequent discarding of defective embryos would avoid the moral dilemma of abortion and the destruction of human beings. The underlying assumption present in that statement needs to be evaluated and challenged. Science has indicated that from the time of conception (when fusion of the maternal and paternal pro-nuclei is complete), the new life (as distinct from mother and father) self-directs its own development with some initial assistance of maternal cytoplasm. In interpreting these scientific facts, many assert that the embryo represents more than a potential person but rather, already, a person with potential. Even if there is yet to be consensus on the interpretation of the scientific facts and the status of the embryo as a person, what does the deliberate destruction of "defective" embryos say to and for children who are born with diseases like Tay-Sachs disease, Duchenne muscular dystrophy, or other birth anomalies? Thus, the protection of new life and the respect that should be accorded to all human beings seems to be lacking in the general discussion of cloning and many reproductive technologies.

Another fundamental issue attached to the technology of cloning is the conceptualization of our relationship with children. In contemporary society, the old maxim that children should be seen and not heard has yielded to a growing phenomenon of physical, sexual, and psychological abuse. In the United States, over one fifth of children live in poverty. Will cloning lead to further insensitivity toward children? Although one must be sensitive to infertile couples, reproductive technologies have suggested in many minds that parents have a right to children. In the process, children take on the status of objects to be possessed rather than subjects to be respected. Certainly, there are many infertile couples who choose *in vitro* fertilization for loving and unselfish reasons. Yet, simultaneously, embryos are discarded because of defects, or in some cases, simply because they are of the wrong sex. Cloning will probably only add to the affront of the dignity of children because couples may have even better means to genetically analyze their child before implantation. The embryos and children take on the semblance of "products" or as one Tennessee divorce case decided, quasi-property. With this strong product metaphor, it is no wonder ethicists are concerned about the development of markets for embryos which would use them as means to an end. On a societal level, one must wonder whether cloning will provide a vehicle in the future for a negative eugenics movement. Although human beings as a whole believe they are beyond such behavior, the xenophobic and ethnic cleansing in Europe should serve as a reminder that a certain unscrupulousness lurks in the depths of the human heart. Moreover, it raises the question about the long range effect on the gene pool and the natural selection process if we select out for certain traits and make multiple copies of people with "desirable" traits.

Test tube twinning may serve to exacerbate already existing problems associated with certain reproductive technologies. Besides the dilemmas associated with famous cases like the Baby M surrogacy case, on a daily basis problems accrue as thousands of embryos today remain frozen in suspended animation, their fate undecided. Cloning will only add to those numbers. In an age of depersonalization of our sexual nature, cloning and asexual reproduction may contribute to the erosion of our sense of the gift of procreativity, of our role as parents, of the meaning of heritage, and of our understanding of sexual intercourse and love. Finally, at a time when our country grapples with ways to provide basic health services to all, is cloning an appropriate and well founded line of investigation when millions of dollars will be devoted to helping only a relatively few number of individuals?

CONCLUSION

In the arena of science and technology, often one is either a technophile or technophobe. Neither position honestly and critically analyzes the advancement of science. To dismiss advances in genetics simply because they draw us closer to a brave new world, denies our creative genius as human beings and our ability to improve our lifestyle. Likewise, to fail to assess the ethical nature and impact of science on humanity would deny the very nature of science itself which necessarily impacts on the human community. A critical assessment of cloning or artificial twinning reveals that it does not involve the exaggerated fears linked to such best sellers as *Jurassic Park*. Nevertheless, the cloning debate has yet to give proper weight to the status of the embryo. Although debate over the embryo will be ongoing, the question we must ask is, can we afford to be wrong when the life of an individual weighs in the balance? Moreover, the applications of cloning reflect an inadequate respect for the developing embryo and an unfortunate movement of viewing the child as object and product rather than personal subject. Even the most innocuous use of cloning—to provide additional embryos to increase the chance of success of pregnancy—should cause us to reflect on the ethical acceptability of various reproductive technologies. As we enter this brave new world of science, society will need insightful women and men of great courage to act on behalf of the human community, especially the children.

NOTE

1. J. Adler, M. Hager, and K. Springen, "Clone Hype," *Newsweek* (November 18, 1993): 61.

63: Baby Theresa: "The Good That Could Be Done"

When Laura Campo and Justin Pearson awaited the birth of their baby, prenatal tests determined early in the pregnancy that the developing fetus suffered from anencephaly, a condition in which the higher centers of the brain fail to develop. Laura and Justin were aware that their baby, when born, would not survive because of this condition. However, they decided to allow the pregnancy to go to term in hopes of donating their baby's organs to other newborns in need of them. When their baby, Theresa, was born, a dispute arose in regard to harvesting her organs.

When an anencephalic infant dies, the cause of death can range from hypoventilation and blood pressure instabilities to endocrine abnormalities and infection.[1] As a result of the manner in which death occurs, the infant's organs may not be suitable for transplantation. Fearing that their baby's organs would be rendered useless if she were allowed to die of natural causes, Theresa's parents sought to have her "declared" dead. Their request was prompted by physicians and others who argued that adhering to the current criteria for determining death causes precious organs to be wasted. But baby Theresa was a living human being because she had a functioning brain stem that maintained integrated human function albeit at a low level. Therefore, the proposal to declare her dead before her brain stem stopped functioning was a proposal to kill her.

It was obvious from the media reports that Theresa's parents were caring persons who neither desired nor intended to harm their child. What, then, prompted such a request? Theresa's parents, like the parents of other anencephalic infants, suffer a great personal tragedy in bearing a child that is "born dying." The desire to find some meaning in the midst of their suffering can lead parents to accept as appropriate the proposal to change the criteria for defining when death has occurred.

The proposal to change the current brain death criteria often reflect one or more of the following assumptions: (1) because the anencephalic infant lacks the capacity for neocortical function the anencephalic infant is not a person; (2) only persons should be considered to be alive and current brain death criteria should be revised to reflect this; (3) using the anencephalic infant's organs for transplantation can "make sense" of a senseless situation; and (4) changing the criteria for determining death would avert the waste of valuable resources that could be used to save the lives of many other infants.

These assumptions will be examined in order to support the conclusion that a) the anencephalic infant is a living human being and should not be killed; b) changing the present criteria for brain death would do nothing to alter the reality of when human death occurs and would serve only to sanction the killing of the infant in order to harvest organs; and c) the desire to temper present suffering should not overcome the ability to make reasoned, ethical decisions about the appropriate care of the anencephalic infant.

ASSESSING THE ASSUMPTIONS

In a utilitarian attempt to maximize the greater good by making more organs available for transplantation, some have argued that the anencephalic infant does not meet the criteria for human personhood. Thus, they maintain that because the cerebral cortex is absent and the infant lacks the capacity for personal activity, the infant should be "declared" dead and the organs harvested. But the lack of present or future capacity for personal activity does not change the fact that the infant is a living human being. The brain stem continues to regulate respiratory and cardiac function. Moreover, "because the neural structures that mediate typical newborn behaviors are located mainly in the brainstem, those anencephalic infants with relatively intact brainstems exhibit many such behaviors."[2]

In addition, attempts to determine a marker event or process (e.g., development of the cerebral cortex) delineating a difference between the human person and the human being consistently have failed.[3] But continued attempts to make such a distinction suggest that for some persons, basic human rights, i.e., the right to life, are understood not to be inherent and inalienable but are, rather, thought to be conferred or earned once certain conditions have been met. One troubling conclusion drawn from this kind of analysis is that the inability to meet the qualifying criteria render our responsibilities to the still living human being null and void. However, reason, supported by medical data, demands that the requirement that death be declared only when the whole brain, i.e., cerebral cortex *and* brain stem, ceases to function should be maintained. And our regard for the still living, though debilitated infant, requires that we refrain from killing regardless of the motivation. In addition, because of the lack of potential for development of higher level functions we should not seek to prolong the anencephalic infant's life by the inappropriate use of life-sustaining interventions.

While this analysis supports the appropriateness of maintaining current brain death criteria, it does nothing to mitigate the suffering experienced by the parents of the anencephalic infant. Nor does it address the appropriateness of trying to "make sense of the tragedy" by changing the rules to allow for killing so as to make the infant's organs available for transplantation. Here, two further considerations are important. First, the desire to overcome the sense of helplessness and hopelessness that accompany the diagnosis and subsequent birth of an anencephalic infant is quite understandable. "These parents want something good to come from their tragedy; they want their child's life to have 'meaning' and the normal and healthy organs of their child to live on."[4] But the meaning or value of human life is not dependent on functional or productive potential. Rather, the good of the human and its meaning are inherent in the human *as* human. This conviction is certainly contrary to the broader societal tendency to assign both personal and social worth commensurate with the ability to produce or contribute to others and/or to society. Second, the proposal to use the infant's organs to help the parents find some measure of solace in their grief shifts the focus of attention from the needs of the dying infant to the needs of the parents. While parental needs are important, the infant is and must remain the primary patient. Appropriate care for the anencephalic infant is to provide those things necessary for comfort and allow death to come. If, after death, organs are adequate for transplantation then they may be used. In addition, the reality of the parents' suffering demands not that the infant be "used" in attempts to "make sense" of their experience. Rather, the parents should be helped to appreciate the inherent good of life, to accept their loss and prepare for the approaching death of their child. Some would argue that such an approach is passive and too readily gives in to the inevitability of death. Rather, such an approach recognizes that human death is a natural part of life and that not every means to overcome the limits associated with human life is consistent with human good or well-being.

Finally, the enthusiasm of those favoring use of the anencephalic's organs for transplantation as a means of saving the lives of other infants must be tempered by reality. Medical data indicates that very few of the anencephalic infants born each year are acceptable as organ donors. But media coverage of cases like baby Theresa's raise false hopes by noting that "about 5,000 children need pediatric organ transplants every year." Such statements are followed by the claim that "anencephalic babies are perfect donors."[5] But nowhere is mention made of the fact that of the estimated 1200 anencephalic infants born each year the usable kidneys, heart and livers are "0, 69 and 61 respectively."[6]

CONCLUSION

The case of baby Theresa raises again issues associated with human suffering, limitation, and death. As we continue to formulate both individual and societal responses to these issues we must keep in mind that expediency should not be allowed to overcome our willingness and ability to make sound ethical and medical judgments. The needs of both the dying infant and the grieving parents require careful and compassionate consideration that aims to promote the good of both.

NOTES

1. D. Alan Shewmon, "Anencephaly: Selected Medical Aspects." *Hastings Center Report* 18 Oct/Nov, 1988, (5): 13.

2. Ibid.

3. President's Commission for the Study of Ethical Problems in Medicine and Research, *Defining Death* (Washington, DC: U.S. Govt. Printing Office, 1981), 39–40.

4. S. Ashwal, et al., "Considerations of Anencephalic Infants as Organ Donor." *Biolaw* 2 (January): 763–69.

5. "Baby Born without Brain Dies, But Legal Struggle Will Continue." *New York Times*, March 31, 1992.

6. D. Alan Shewmon, et. al., "The Use of Anencephalic Infants as Organ Sources," *JAMA* 261 (12): 1774.

64: The Baby Fae Legacy

Baby Fae was the first infant to receive a transplant of a baboon heart. Although she lived just short of three weeks with the transplant, the medical treatment she received spawned a host of ethical questions that live after her. We shall consider some of these questions in this essay.

PRINCIPLES

When doing research involving human subjects, most physicians and scientists in the United States follow regulations for ethical research published by agencies of the federal government. Indeed, if the research in question is funded by the federal government, following the federal regulations is mandatory. Evaluating human research protocols to ensure conformity with federal regulations is the responsibility of the institutional review board (IRB). An IRB, required at every research institution, is mainly concerned with protecting the human subjects involved in research projects, but has some concern with the scientific validity of the project as well. At some schools, Saint Louis University, for example, all research projects involving human subjects must be approved by the IRB, not only those funded by the federal government.

The federal regulations for research involving children envision two types of research: that which "holds out prospects of direct benefit for the individual subject" and that which "does not hold out the prospect of direct benefit for the individual subject."[1] In this latter type of research, there may be a benefit resulting from the study, such as new scientific knowledge, that would benefit other children, but there is no direct benefit for the child or children involved in the research project. Concerning the first type of research that involves therapeutic treatment for the child or children in question, the regulations for ethical research are similar to those regulating research on adult human subjects. Hence, consent must be received (in this case proxy consent, because the child cannot give informed consent) and the risk of harm envisioned must be justified by the anticipated benefit.

In regard to the research on children who do not benefit directly, however, the regulations are more involved.

First, a distinction is made between "minimal risk of harm" to the subject and "more than minimal risk of harm." *Minimal risk* is equivalent to "physical and psychological harm that is normally encountered in the daily lives or in the routine medical or psychological examination of healthy children." Research that involves "*more than* minimal risk" may be approved by the IRB

219

if there is "only a *minor increase* over minimal risk" and other requirements are met. If the IRB finds that the research involves a *major increase* over minimal risk, "the IRB can refer the project to the Department of Health and Human Services for study by a panel of experts," provided the IRB also "finds that the research presents a reasonable opportunity to further the understanding, prevention or alleviation of a serious problem affecting the health and welfare of children."

Some ethicists, ourselves included, believe the federal regulations for *Research Involving Children* are too lenient insofar as nonbeneficial research is concerned. The main reason for this disagreement lies in the nature of proxy consent. A parent or guardian has the right of proxy consent only in order to benefit his or her child or ward. Although an adult may freely subject himself or herself to risk research in which there is no personal benefit, it seems that a parent or guardian does not have the same right over a child. Whatever the value of this opinion, it seems that the treatment given Baby Fae was unethical even if evaluated in light of the more liberal ethical norms contained in the federal regulations.

DISCUSSION

In order to offer an ethical evaluation, let us ask the following questions:

1. Should the physicians who performed the transplant on Baby Fae follow the federal guidelines for research on children? Legally speaking, they did not have to follow these guidelines because the research was funded by withholding a portion of the fees collected from private patients. (This method of funding research is an ethical issue in itself because cost shifting is involved.) Morally speaking, though, it seems that the researchers at Loma Linda University do have an obligation to follow the federal regulations because they offer minimal ethical standards for our pluralistic society. To put it another way, if researchers do not follow the federal norms, which ethical norms will they follow?

2. Did this research benefit Baby Fae directly or did it offer the kind of knowledge that would benefit other children? Despite some early enthusiastic statements from some of the physicians doing the transplant, there seems to be no doubt that the transplant was not of direct benefit to Baby Fae. Some might say, "Baby Fae benefited because she would have died anyway and the transplant prolonged her life." But research may never be justified simply because the subject "will die anyway." Moreover, what benefit is it to prolong the life of an infant for three weeks and treat the infant as a thing rather than a person during that time? Others might say, "Maybe by some miracle

she could have lived." But scientific research on human beings is not based on miracles, it is based on certified knowledge and previous research on animals. To say that the research did not benefit Baby Fae directly does not imply it was per se unethical, but it does mean that such research should be subject to stringent standards.

3. If the research did not benefit Baby Fae, did it involve more than minimal risk of harm? If so, was it a minor or a major increase? Clearly the surgery involved a major risk of harm. Not only was there the risk of immediate death, but there was the certainty of physical pain and suffering from the surgery and of deterioration of vital organs from the drugs used to suppress Baby Fae's immunological defenses. In addition to the risk of physical harm, the risk of emotional harm must be considered as well. Baby Fae spent her last days as a research object, not in the arms of a loving mother. In sum, it seems that the IRB at Loma Linda University did not have the right to approve the research on Baby Fae.

CONCLUSION

Because there was no hope of benefiting Baby Fae and because the risk of harm involved in the transplant procedure was a major increase over minimal harm, it seems that the baboon heart research proposal should have been submitted to a national panel of experts selected by the Secretary of Health and Human Services. Research involving transplants from animals is not in itself unethical, but it should be carried on only after the protocol, its scientific justification, and an analysis of risk and benefit have been evaluated and approved by a group of competent peers.

NOTE

1. *Research Involving Children* (Washington, DC: National Commission for Protection of Human Subjects of Biomedical and Behavioral Research, OS77–0004, 1977); *Federal Register* vol. 48, n. 46 (Washington, DC: U.S. Government Printing Office, March 8, 1983); "Additional Protection for Children Involved as Subjects of Research," *Federal Register*, vol. 48, n. 46 (Washington, DC: U.S. Government Printing Office, March 8, 1983).

65: "Only God Can Heal My Daughter"

Twelve-year-old Pamela Hamilton broke her leg. When treating her broken leg, her physician discovered a cancerous tumor, which was diagnosed as Ewing's sarcoma. Larry Hamilton, Pamela's father and pastor at the Church of God of the Union Assembly, La Follette, Tennessee, and her mother, Deborah, refused treatment of Pamela's cancer because taking medicine is against their religion. "Only God can heal my daughter," declared her father: "She has the faith to recover; it will be God's will if she does not." Having been notified of Pamela's condition, the Tennessee Department of Social Service petitioned the courts for custody of Pamela on the grounds that her life was endangered because of her parents' religious beliefs. By the time the courts of Tennessee granted the transfer of custody, two months had elapsed. The attending physician stated that she had only a fifty percent chance of survival because of the "red hot and angry tumor which now has spread through her thigh and up to the hip joint." Even though her life was endangered, Pamela agreed with her parent's decision and declared, "I do not want radiation and chemotherapy because I do not want my hair to fall out or to be sick."

PRINCIPLES

When considering the relationship between parents and children from the Judeo-Christian ethical perspective, two interrelated assumptions are paramount. First the family unit must be fostered and protected because it is the fundamental element on which society and culture depend for strength and continuity. Second, parents should have care and custody of their children because experience shows that parents love their children and strive to help them become virtuous human beings. Like most ethical assumptions, this latter one yields to contrary evidence. Hence, if parents are abusing their children and endangering their lives, then society intervenes and removes the children from the parents' custody, at least for a time. The right of intervention on behalf of children illustrates another ethical assumption; namely, that parents do not "own" their children. Rather, parents are stewards, caretakers, of their children, enablers who help their children grow in knowledge and virtue. Above all, life and death decisions concerning children are not to be made for the parents' benefit.

    Both ethical reasoning and legal precedent give priority to the expression of a person's religious faith. Because religious faith is the most personal, important, and profound act of conscience, its expression should not be limited unless it is manifestly injurious to other people. Hence, as long as parents respect the well-being of their children, they have the ethical and legal right to rear and educate their children in the religion of the parents' choice. The right to choose a religion for children, as well as many other rights, gradually wanes as children mature and are able to make competent decisions for themselves. Here, of course, we encounter the crux of the matter: When are children able to make competent decisions for themselves? When do children become young adults? The laws of every country try to solve this question by stating that, for legal purposes, young people become adults at age 17, 18, or 21, depending on the right in question. (Strangely, in most states, young people may marry at an earlier age than they may buy alcoholic beverages.) The laws, however, express only a general norm; it may often happen that a young person is mature enough to make important decisions for himself or herself well before the legal age of maturity. In recognition of this fact, ethicists now suggest that capable children be asked to give their "assent" to surgery or other serious medical treatments, even though the proxy consent of their parents or guardian will suffice for ethical and legal clearance for medical treatment.

DISCUSSION

Cases resembling that of Pamela Hamilton are not unusual. The courts frequently appoint guardians for children whose parents, being Jehovah's Witnesses, believe that the Bible prohibits blood transfusions even when death would occur without them. The ethical basis for court action is the assumption that the child's life should not be endangered by the parent's religious beliefs. Even if the child agrees with the parents' belief, the ethical and legal thinking in most of these cases is that the child cannot make a competent decision and, because life is such as important gift, that he or she would choose life if a competent and free decision were possible.

Pamela's situation is different from the usual transfer of custody case for religious reasons. First, she agrees with her parents' decision that she should not receive medicine for treatment of cancer. On the face of it, the parent's statement that "God will cure" is rather unreasonable. Although religious people attribute omnipotence to God and, in that sense, believe that God does cure, they usually do not deny that human beings have a cooperative role to fulfill in effecting a cure. That human beings will one day die is assured, but they have a right and a duty to use positive means such as medicine and surgery to prolong their lives as long as living enables them to pursue the goal of life. But even though the belief of Pamela and her parents seems unreasonable, it is a religious belief and should be honored unless it manifestly harms other people.

This brings us to the second issue that makes Pamela's case somewhat different: there was a threat that she would die within a year even if chemotherapy and radiation were used. The fact that she might survive does not obviate the need for the court to question at the time of the original discussion: What if we take her from her family, give her extensive chemotherapy, and she dies anyway?

In most states, if Pamela were over 18 and stated that because of her religious beliefs she did not wish to receive medical treatment for her tumor, people might try to persuade her to change her mind, but, in the last analysis, they would be legally and ethically bound to respect her decision. The question that bothers is: Even though she is only twelve years old, did the court make an effort to determine her maturity? No doubt Pamela's faith is strong, but is it due to her parents' influence or to her own free convictions? And did the court consider the gravity of her condition before making its decision?

CONCLUSION

Given the choice, most people will choose life over death, and legal precedent must be based on what happens most of the time. But legal precedent alone does not guarantee an ethical solution. In order to have an ethical solution, legal precedent must be interpreted in light of the pertinent facts of the case and the ethical assumptions on which the precedent is based. Pamela's case reminds us that religious and family rights are very important and that the courts must consider particular facts and assumptions as well as precedent in order to form ethical decisions.

Note: Fourteen-year-old Pamela Hamilton died from cancer one year after being taken from the care of her parents. Although Pamela received treatment and her cancer was considered in remission for awhile, the therapy was ultimately ineffective.

66: Treatment of Rape Victims

Two recent events bring the question of ethical treatment of rape victims into consideration. First, the development of a true "morning after pill," RU486, an extremely effective method of terminating pregnancy within the first nine weeks of gestation. Second, an appellate court in California ruled that Catholic hospitals have the responsibility "to provide information concerning, and access to, estrogen prophylaxis for rape victims." Since the court case involved Catholic hospitals, this essay will consider the proper treatment of rape victims from the perspective of Catholic teaching.

PRINCIPLES

A victim of rape should be given the most sensitive and charitable care possible. Victims often complain justifiably that they are treated, by the police and medical personnel alike, as though they were responsible for provoking the attack, thus compounding the grave injustice from which the woman has suffered. Hospital procedures for treatment of rape victims should be designed to accomplish four things:

1. To offer the psychological support and counseling that the woman needs to work through the trauma of the attack and its aftermath.
2. To provide medical care for injuries or abrasions that might have occurred.
3. To gather evidence to be used if the rapist is apprehended and prosecuted.
4. To provide treatment to prevent possible venereal disease and pregnancy.

This last point, preventing pregnancy, raises special ethical problems. Avoiding pregnancy is a very serious concern for a rape victim and she deserves every help that medical professionals can give, provided that help is ethical. In many cases, it will be possible to determine that conception is not feasible, for example, if the woman is taking contraceptive drugs or if an examination of cervical mucus shows she is not in a fertile phase. If pregnancy is a possibility, however, since the victim is in no way responsible for the possible pregnancy, she has the right to avoid conception. A woman who has consented to intercourse takes responsibility as a free person to use the sexual act in keeping with its intrinsic significance of love and procreation.

The rape victim has no such responsibility because she has not consented to the sexual act. Once a woman has conceived, however, she cannot take any direct action to abort or to destroy a fertilized ovum or request others to do so. Because a fertilized ovum is a human being, albeit in incipient stage, it deserves the respect due human life. Ethical problems arise, then, when methods to prevent conception are utilized that may have the effect of preventing conception, but that also may cause the destruction of a fertilized ovum if conception has already occurred.

DISCUSSION

In the United States, most hospital rape protocols recommend the administration of antifertility drugs such as Ovral in large dosage (100 mlg.) within seventy-two hours of the rape; a second dose being taken twelve hours later. The rape protocols specify that Ovral or other estrogenic hormones should not be administered until a test is given to determine if the woman is pregnant. If the pregnancy test is positive, the pregnancy occurred before the rape and treatment with Ovral may injure the embryo.

May rape protocols that call for the administration of Ovral be utilized in a Catholic hospital? Ovral and similar estrogenic compounds have two effects: they inhibit ovulation, but they also impede implantation of the embryo if fertilization has already occurred. Hence, if Ovral is given with the intention of inhibiting ovulation and preventing conception, its use is acceptable, provided it is given at a time in the woman's cycle when it could prevent ovulation, or impede the motility of the sperm, and thus prevent fertilization. Hence, any antifertility medication must be given within seventy-two hours of the rape. Otherwise, the effect of the medication would be useless in preventing conception because the sperm would be inactive or dead. If the antiovulatory medication is given at a time in the menstrual cycle when its only effect would be to prevent implantation of the fertilized ovum, then its use would not be acceptable. The principle of double effect justifies the use of Ovral or similar medications if the intention is to avoid conception and the medication is given at a time in the woman's cycle when ovulation has not occurred.

What if there is doubt as to whether or not the woman has ovulated, a situation that would be true of many women who present themselves for treatment after rape. A Catholic ethics committee in Great Britain asked this question and responded, rightly it seems, that if there is doubt as to whether ovulation has occurred within the present menstrual cycle, antifertility drugs may be used with the intention of preventing ovulation because the probability that fertilization has occurred is minimal.[1] The doubt in question concerns the fact of ovulation, not the fact of conception.

Notice that Ovral and other estrogenic hormones that inhibit ovulation are entirely different from RU486, the true "morning after pill." When used after intercourse, RU486 has *only* an abortifacient effect. RU486 produces its effect by blocking the normal action of the hormone progesterone, thus preventing implantation of the fertilized ovum. Hence, in care for rape victims, RU486, the true "morning after pill," is not an alternative for Catholic hospitals. At present, RU486 is sold commercially only in France and China; how long it will be unavailable in other countries is a question. Much confusion has been generated by courts, lawyers, and health care professionals who use the term "morning after pill" to refer to medications that are utilized with the intention of preventing conception. A firm distinction should be made between antiovulatory medications, such as Ovral, and RU486.

CONCLUSION

What is the import of the decision of the California appeals court insofar as Catholic hospitals are concerned? First, the California court declared the responsibility of the hospital to provide "information concerning, and access to, estrogen pregnancy prophylaxis" for rape victims. It allowed the hospital to fulfill this responsibility "by instructing the patient concerning the options for pregnancy prevention and by transferring the patient to another medical facility or another physician." However, it seems Catholic hospitals are justified in offering direct service to rape victims. Hence, every Catholic hospital should have an explicit policy that delineates the circumstances in which antifertility medications may be used to help rape victims avoid conception. Second, the concept of abortion put forward by the California appeals court is not acceptable from the perspective of Catholic teaching. The court considers efforts to prevent implantation of a fertilized ovum to be "birth control," while Catholic teaching considers this to be abortion. A better effort to present to the court the scientific evidence maintaining that a fertilized ovum is a human being, even before implantation, seems to be in order.

NOTE

1. "Use of the Morning After Pill in Rape Cases." *Origins*, March 13, 1986: 633.

Note: Using medication to prevent ovulation in proper circumstances is also supported by a recent statement of the Pennsylvania Catholic Conference. (*Origins*, Vol. 22, No.47, May 6, 1993, p. 81).

67: Kevorkian's Dilemma: Are We Owners or Stewards of Human Life?

Dr. Jack Kevorkian strikes again. Kevorkian, the retired pathologist who designed a death machine, has assisted at least 19 people to commit suicide. The actions of Kevorkian have evoked criticism and even outrage from people in the medical, legal, and ethical professions, as well as from leaders of religious communities. On the other hand, many seem to agree with him.

In a certain sense there is a logic in Kevorkian's efforts to assist people to commit suicide. Anyone who subscribes to the interpretation of autonomy favored by some legal decisions in the United States will find some meaning in the Kevorkian death machine. This legal interpretation is founded in the oft-quoted dictum of former Supreme Court Justice Benjamin Cardozo, "Every human being of adult years and sound mind has the right to determine what will be done with his own body."

Cardozo's dictum is rooted radically in Enlightenment thinking, and is best expressed in the writings of John Locke who looked upon the state merely as a vehicle for protecting individual rights. Not irrationally, Justice Cardozo's dictum has been interpreted by many legal experts and ethicists to indicate that human beings have absolute dominion over their bodies and thus their lives, in the same way that they would have dominion over a piece of property.

Just as persons may use, sell, or even destroy a car or a suit of clothing as it pleases them, so persons have the same power over their bodies and thus their lives. According to this view of human life and freedom, suicide becomes a "right," and if a person needs assistance in committing suicide, then there is a "right" to the assistance that is needed. While the words of Cardozo originally were used to demonstrate the need for informed consent before invasive medical procedures were performed, it does not take much imagination to use them in defense of suicide and assisted suicide.

Opposed to this concept of absolute dominion over body and life is a concept that envisions persons as stewards or caretakers of their bodies and of their lives. Stewardship recognizes the power of the person to make free decisions designed to achieve the goods and goals of life. But stewardship also posits that there are goods and goals of life that are innate. Indeed, the most fundamental and important goods and goals of life are innate.

To put it another way, the stewardship concept of the human person assumes that our drive toward worshiping God, respecting life as a gift,

228

honoring one's parents, and striving for happiness, self-esteem, friendship, creativity, truth, and longevity arise from our very nature. Our Constitution codified these innate goods and goals as "life, liberty, and the pursuit of happiness." These and other significant objectives toward which we direct our affections and actions result from the fact that we are not free to choose or reject the basic goals of life. Accordingly, in the stewardship view of the human person, killing oneself has always been considered a harmful action because it makes it impossible to strive for the basic goods of life.

The concept of stewardship is founded not merely in religious teaching or in mythology. Rather, it proceeds from an understanding that each person has innate goods and goals for which he or she strives, and that some actions are helpful in achieving these goals, and other actions are detrimental insofar as achieving these goals are concerned. Killing innocent people, for example, has been rejected as incompatible with the goods and goals of life. Nourishing and caring for infants has always been considered as an act fulfilling the goods and goals of life. This view of the person, his or her moral responsibilities, and the rejection of suicide and assisted suicide have been much more accepted in Western society than the opposite attitude. If the view of a person as owner of his body and life is so opposed to the view that has been traditional in Western society, why do so many people support the efforts of Dr. Kevorkian and why is there a waiting list for use of his suicide device? Why did the dictum of Cardozo take so long to surface as a justification for suicide and assisted suicide? Why is there a tendency today to accept suicide and physician-assisted suicide, when accepting these actions would have been unthinkable twenty years ago?

Though several factors in our society contribute to acceptance of suicide and assisted suicide as legal and ethical options, the following factors seem most significant.

First, our society is characterized by the philosophy of individualism as opposed to communitarianism. Individualism leads us to think that our well-being and self-worth depend upon our ability "to take care of ourselves." Individualism not only teaches us to depend on our own resources exclusively, but tends to make us think that we are bad people, or social failures if we must depend upon others. How often do we hear people say, "I don't want to be a burden to others"? Faced with "being a burden" or suicide, some under the influence of individualism will opt for suicide. Often, there may be many people in a person's family or social unit capable of rendering compassionate help, but the help is not accepted because the individualistic person, even when suffering, habitually rejects the help of others. Expecting an aging or chronically ill person to be independent and "not a burden" is as foolish as expecting a newborn baby to be independent and "not a burden." Sometimes acknowledging dependence is a very natural and beneficial recognition.

Second, self-worth in our society is assumed to depend upon the individual's ability to contribute to economic productivity. In a more communitarian view of the person, worth and value of the individual are based upon one's human nature. With this view of those who can no longer contribute actively as economic factors in society, depression and despair are avoided through compassionate care of suffering people.

Finally, many people are disposed to choose suicide because they fear losing control of their lives as death approaches, and thus are tempted to choose suicide as a means of exercising control of their lives. Specifically, people who envision death, especially those in pain, fear their lives will be prolonged through medical therapy that is not truly beneficial. Moreover, they fear that their pain will not be controlled. While both of these fears have some basis in reality, efforts to overcome both aberrations of medical practice are being addressed in medical schools and residency programs. Because of American medicine's unquestioning acceptance of technology, the tendency to overtreat patients as death approaches will be more difficult to overcome than the undertreatment of pain. The acceptance granted Kevorkian's plan and the tendency of some physicians to help their patient commit suicide are symptoms of a profession that at present is not able to handle death in an ennobling and supportive manner.

Depending upon the way in which one views human responsibility, one will accept or reject suicide and physician-assisted suicide as an ethical choice. Are we owners or stewards of human life? If we are owners of human life, then humans set their own standards for right and wrong behavior. But with this exaggerated view of human dominion, ethics becomes a word game, society a jungle, and each person becomes ruler of his or her own world as Niechtze predicted. On the other hand, if we are stewards of body and life, our fulfillment consists in striving for the goods and goals of life, the most important of which are innate.

68: Nightmare of the "Living Dead"

Physicians pronounce a young boy dead by means of whole brain death criteria (the irreversible loss of cortical and brain stem function). However, the family, in a state of denial, demands that "life support" be continued indefinitely. Litigation ensues and the court ultimately sides with the physicians and orders support to be withdrawn. Unfortunately, such a scenario of inappropriate family requests surfaces more commonly than expected. This in part results from the general public's perception that "brain death" means permanent unconsciousness rather than human death. Studies indicate that health care professionals also lack clarity over the meaning and concept of brain death. Consequently, this misunderstanding coupled with a tendency of health care professionals to use brain death as a criterion for assessing the use or nonuse of life sustaining interventions has led to conflict. This essay will focus on the issue of dealing with a family that refuses to stop "life support" after death. How can clinicians be tactful and compassionate to grieving relatives while avoiding the ceding of their responsibility to an exaggerated and inappropriate understanding of family rights?

PRINCIPLES

Traditionally in health care, physicians determined death by the irreversible cessation of circulatory and respiratory function. With the advent of complex life-support technology, even though a person's whole brain had ceased functioning, respiration and blood circulation could be maintained artificially for a certain period of time, although usually for no more than a week before the body would begin to decay. These advances in technology necessitated a new manner for assessing death while vital functions were maintained in the hope of removing organs for transplant. In the late 1960s, Harvard Medical School published the Harvard criteria, which provided a means to determine whether a patient whose heart and respiration were maintained artificially was indeed dead. It involved both a physical exam and confirmatory electroencephalogram evidence. Subsequently, scientists developed brain blood flow studies to facilitate the determination of brain death. People initially harbored some misgivings about the criteria, fearing that transplant teams would remove organs from living patients. Now, with the exception of a few cultures, whole brain death has become an acceptable standard for determining death. However, with the

231

passage of time, brain death has been used more frequently as a criterion for the removal of "life support." Consequently, like other cases where families demand futile treatments over the objection of the health care team, families also have insisted that brain dead loved ones continue to be treated. How should health care workers respond to such requests?

The inherent purpose of health care is to treat the living whether that involves curing patients, helping them live with disabilities, or keeping them comfortable as death approaches. Once death has been determined, support should be removed unless the family has chosen to donate organs. In fact, the physician has a positive obligation to remove support, to do otherwise would squander health care resources whether that be on a micro level (e.g., the critical care bed), or on a macro level (e.g., valuable health care dollars and resources that would serve only to continue to add to the high price of health care). Justice demands a judicious use of resources. Common sense dictates that one does not make a practice of perfusing a corpse. However, this intellectual conviction often falls prey to distraught family members who demand continued treatment for their brain dead loved one for a variety of reasons ranging from a denial of death to suspicion of the health care profession.

DISCUSSION

Knowing the right thing to do often does not coincide with doing the right thing. Yet, ethics in health care demands not only the knowing but also the doing. Certain factors arise in the professional setting that inhibit one from doing the right thing. This results in families holding the health care team hostage resulting in a corpse being "kept alive." What are some of those factors?

First, the dominance of individualism and consumerism in health care decision making leaves the impression that clinicians have a duty to do whatever the family or patient wants regardless of the request, especially if it does no harm to someone else. However, the health care professional/patient relationship only requires that potentially beneficial treatments be offered to patients. Thus, physicians should not acquiesce to requests to "maintain corpses." To do so merely relegates the physician to the role of technician. Second, clinicians fear lawsuits from vocal families of patients who refuse to allow life support to be removed from brain dead individuals. Although there would be no basis for a lawsuit by the family, practitioners and hospital lawyers sometimes choose the path of least resistance and perfuse a corpse rather than face a potential lawsuit. In the short run, this may bypass conflict and bad publicity, but in the long run, it distorts what health care is about and reinforces a faulty notion of autonomy in the minds of people. Third, a misplaced sense of compassion may tempt clinicians to continue life support for the deceased because a family is in a state of denial especially if death resulted from sudden trauma. This situation can be further complicated if the clinician feels uncomfortable about dealing with issues of death and dying with families. Therefore, rather than remove support, physicians may believe that they should continue to maintain the corpse to spare the family the pain of acceptance of death until they are ready. Clinicians may argue that we make exceptions for perfusing a corpse for the sake of others (e.g., organ recipients), then why not do so to lessen the emotional pain of a family having a hard time coming to grips with the death of a loved one. Unfortunately, this may serve only to further the impression that the patient is still alive; otherwise, why would the doctors still be treating the patient if there were not some hope? Nor does this embody a healthy approach to dealing with denial while valuable ICU resources and monies are wasted. Consequently, although doctors may allow families time to say good-bye to loved ones, they should not delay the removal of interventions for any undue length of time. Fourth, families may be reluctant to allow for the removal of support because they believe that the physicians are declaring death prematurely in order to harvest organs. This concern should not be overlooked. Studies of organ donation patterns cite this concern as a major reason for failure to donate organs. Thus, health care professionals making requests for organs should be distinct from those involved in patient care. This will reduce the appearance of a conflict of interests. Fifth, after brain death, statements from care givers like "we'll remove life support now and allow the patient to die," serve only to confuse families. Therefore, care givers should be clear and accurate in their understanding of brain death lest they unknowingly distress families. Sixth, families of certain cultural or religious backgrounds may reject whole brain death as an acceptable definition of death. In some states the law has recognized this right of conscience. Yet this right does not imply a corresponding obligation for clinicians to fulfill requests that are inconsistent with the tenets of ethics and medicine. Physicians incur no responsibility to provide an absolutely futile treatment as understood by the medical profession. Finally, sometimes clinicians utilize brain death as a criterion for determining whether to continue life-sustaining interventions. Perhaps the use of brain death as a criterion for removing life support is indicative of a discomfort about withdrawing life support from patients before death occurs because of personal or legal concerns. However, less complicated and less expensive tools of assessment are available for this purpose. Ironically, the use of brain death as a criterion for removing life support at times has led to unreasonable demands by families to continue to perfuse a corpse.

Ethical and sensitive management of brain death cases can be achieved when health care professionals recognize and cope appropriately with the preceding factors. Communication must be clear and family members should be queried in order to ensure they understand the nature of the situation.

Often, in layman's parlance, "brain dead" refers to what medically speaking constitutes a persistent vegetative state. Family members must understand that "brain death" means the patient is dead, not just in an irreversible coma. In fact, clinicians may choose to avoid the term altogether in order to avoid confusion. Physicians should also request the aid of appropriate services (pastoral care, social work, psychiatry) from the onset to deal with any issues of denial of death.

CONCLUSION

Sound communication, patience, and sympathy can help to defuse some of the emotionally charged issues associated with brain death. Nevertheless, through no fault of their own, health care workers encounter families who remain adamant in their requests to continue to perfuse a corpse. Clinicians may be tempted to follow the directives of families. Yet, to do so simply may result in bad medicine. Besides providing the family with a false sense of hope, continued support also violates the norms of justice and appropriate stewardship of the goods of health care. More important, it perverts the role of the clinician as a trained professional with expertise. Although one would want to try to avoid an adversarial position wherein families threaten lawsuits, physicians and, more importantly, administrators should stand firm in their conviction in the face of lawsuits of such frivolous merit. Clinicians who know they have the backing of the institution's administration in making ethical decisions will be much more likely not only to know the right thing to do, but to do it as well.

Dealing with the families of brain dead patients can be taxing and frustrating at times. Many problems can be obviated by not using brain death as a criterion for removing life support. Rather it should be used to verify a patient's death before organ removal. When families request that life support be continued after death for whatever reasons, clinicians should hold fast to what they know is ethically right. To do otherwise in the long run only will subvert the nature of the health care profession and do a disservice to the patient's family and the rest of society.

69: Anencephaly and the Management of Pregnancy

The ethical assessment of human actions must be based on appropriate data and guided by a process of reasoned analysis. The precision demanded by this process depends on both conceptual and linguistic exactness in order to describe and analyze accurately what is at issue. This is particularly true when contemplating decisions and actions involving human life and death. In this arena, ongoing ethical analysis may yield new conclusions as the pertinent data changes in light of developments in medicine, technology, and the like. Such developments make it possible to gain more accuracy in both describing and understanding the reality at hand as well as in evaluating contemplated actions relative to that reality. In this essay, I will explore the effects that the ability to diagnose anencephaly very early in pregnancy *may* have on the ethical analysis of the management of the pregnancy.

At present, when a woman is known to be carrying an anencephalic fetus, many conscientious physicians and couples reject early delivery as an option. Rather, they choose to wait until the fetus reaches the stage of viability before inducing labor to end the pregnancy. Upon delivery, the anencephalic newborn is given only comfort care and is allowed to die. This practice is consistent with the belief that any intervention to terminate pregnancy *before* viability constitutes a *direct* abortion. Such actions are immoral. This view is expressed in the *Ethical and Religious Directives for Catholic Health Facilities*. "Abortion, that is, the directly intended termination of pregnancy before viability, is never permitted."[1] But an intervention that is directed at the cure of a proportionately serious pathological condition of the mother can be made before viability even though the fetus may die as a result. Because the immediate purpose of the intervention is to cure the pathology the resulting fetal death is *indirect*.

The evaluation yielding this conclusion is guided by the principle of double effect. This principle serves to ensure two things in the analysis of actions having both good and evil effects. First, one must not intend or do that which is evil even in the pursuit of good. Second, one should prevent any evil, even indirect, from occurring insofar as it is possible to do so. Accordingly, an action taken having both good and evil effects must be good or morally indifferent. The good outcome must be the direct effect and the evil outcome merely permitted. Note that if the good can be achieved without causing the evil effect, the evil must be avoided. Finally, in order to permit

235

the evil as an indirect result, the good intended by the action must be of due proportion. Thus, allowing for the death of a fetus for an insignificant reason would be ethically indefensible. But the adequacy of the proportion between the good intended and the evil allowed is a matter of prudential judgment. Such a judgment is not a matter of mere opinion. Rather, it must be informed by appropriate factual data and be the result of careful consideration.

Can this kind of analysis be applied to the case of the previable anencephalic fetus? The question is raised because of the ability to diagnose anencephaly as early as the first trimester of pregnancy and the realization that, once the diagnosis is made, there seems to be no purpose in maintaining the pregnancy.

MEDICAL DATA

Anencephaly is a condition in which major portions of the brain, skull, and scalp are congenitally absent. The incidence of anencephaly is from 0.6 to 3.5 per 1,000 births[2] and results from failure of the neural tube to close early in the process of embryonic development. The condition can be diagnosed in the first trimester of pregnancy. Diagnosis is based upon elevated levels of maternal serum alpha-fetoprotein and is confirmed by high-resolution ultrasonography.[3] In pregnancies that go to term the newborn lacks a functioning cerebral cortex and, as a result, has no capacity to develop cognitive-affective function. The condition is uniformly fatal, death usually occurring hours after birth from cardiorespiratory arrest.

Pregnancy with an anencephalic fetus can put the mother at increased risk. "Labor and delivery are commonly associated with unstable fetal lie, dysfunctional labor and postpartum hemorrhage."[4] Moreover, the emotional trauma suffered by a couple upon diagnosis of anencephaly understandably can be considerable.

DISCUSSION

Pregnancy is a process that begins when sperm and ovum unite to form a new human life. The goal of this process is to provide the necessary environment in which that new life can grow and develop in an integrated manner. If the process proceeds normally over its developmental course, the result will be a live born infant having the capacity for continued, integrated growth and development. Because we are discussing *human* development appropriate understanding of the concept of integration is essential. The emphasis on integration derives from the fact that human life, while dependent upon a physiologic substrate, involves psychologic, social, and creative capacities as well. In other words, human life involves more than simply biologic life. The organ responsible and essential for the integration of the levels of function characteristic of human life is the brain, specifically the cerebral cortex. But it is the cerebral cortex that is absent in anencephaly. As a result, only physiologic development can occur and that only in a limited way. Once the defect occurs, integrated development is no longer possible. Thus, the anencephalic fetus has reached its human developmental potential and maintaining pregnancy serves only to preserve limited physiologic growth. It is only in light of an adequate understanding of the concept of integration that the notion of viability can be considered. Viability is a quality acquired by the already living fetus during the process of pregnancy. It indicates the ability of the fetus to continue to live, grow and develop *on its own* outside the uterus. But anencephaly makes integrated development impossible. Thus, the living but previable fetus is developmentally complete in terms of human development once the defect responsible for anencephaly expresses itself. The anencephalic fetus can never acquire the quality of viability, appropriately understood, and thus viability has no meaning as a moral marker in such cases.

CONCLUSIONS

On the basis of the above analysis it seems that once the diagnosis of anencephaly has been made the pregnancy may be terminated at any time. While there is no life-threatening maternal pathology, the mother is at risk because of the fetal pathology. The intervention that terminates the pregnancy is taken to avoid the continued risk to the mother posed by carrying an anencephalic fetus. The risks cannot be averted in any other way. The death of the fetus, while unintended, is unavoidable. It is a matter of prudential judgment that the good being sought in this case is of due proportion to the evil permitted. While the mother's life is not in imminent danger, there is the real possibility of maternal harm as pregnancy advances. Since the condition of the fetus deprives it of any potential for development, the proportion seems adequate to justify terminating the pregnancy. Moreover, because of its condition the anencephalic fetus, though living from the moment of conception, will never achieve viability.

The importance of maintaining appropriate regard for nascent human life cannot be overstated. This is particularly true in a society that seems to have lost much of its reverence for life. But concern to preserve appropriate respect for life must not curtail thoughtful, ongoing critical analysis of issues when new information raises questions about the adequacy of prior judgments.

NOTES

1. United States Catholic Conference, *Ethical and Religious Directives for Catholic Health Facilities*, Directive #12.

2. D. K. Kalousek, et al., *Pathology of the Human Embryo and Previable Fetus* (London: Springer-Verlag, 1990).

3. David Nyberg, M.D., et al., *Diagnostic Ultrasound of Fetal Anomalies* (Chicago: Year Book Medical Publishers, Inc.: 1990), 146–52.

4. Medical Task Force on Anencephaly, "The Infant with Anencephaly," *New England Journal of Medicine* 322 (10).

70: HIV Testing for Health Care Workers: Has Its Time Come?

In early May of 1993, health officials identified a sixth patient who had contracted HIV infection from Florida dentist David Acer. In the wake of this latest revelation, the public reissued demands for mandatory testing of health care professionals. Public opinion polls consistently indicate that over 90 percent of those polled want to know the HIV status of their physicians. Patient advocate groups citing the necessity that patients be fully informed of the risks of a procedure, insist that patients must have access to the HIV status of health care professionals in order to make true informed consent. In response, health care associations have opposed vehemently any type of mandatory testing or disclosure because of the minuscule probability of transmission of infection from health care worker to patient. They cite as a particular concern the destructive potential of revealing the HIV status of the health care professional. This essay will explore the highly charged debate to determine whether mandatory testing and disclosure would benefit all parties involved or merely perpetuate overreaction to a disease that frequently has engendered irrational and exaggerated fears.

PRINCIPLES

Ethical analysis requires sound medical facts on which to base its conclusion. While transmission of HIV infection from patient to health care worker via occupational exposure to infected fluids has been well documented, it has been infrequent. The possibility of transmission in the other direction is lower. Whereas the health care worker may be exposed to large amounts of a patient's infected blood, the patient is exposed to only a minimal amount of the infected blood of the health care worker, thus reducing the possibility of contagion. So far, the only documented incident of infection passing from health care professional to patients has been the case of the Florida dentist. However, the uncertainty surrounding the mode of transmission, the emerging evidence that the dentist may have infected his patients intentionally, and the clustering of cases have combined to raise doubts about viewing this case as a valid physician-patient transmission. Retrospective studies of transmission from infected physicians to patients appearing in *JAMA* (April 14, 1993) reveal no incidents of transmission. Although look-back studies have inherent limitations, specifically that some patients may not choose to be tested, still the data should have a determinative role in deciding the appropriateness of mandatory testing. Statistically, when the HIV status of a surgeon is unknown, the risk of infection to the patient is estimated to be 1 in 21 million per hour of surgery. If the surgeon is HIV infected, the estimate of the risk still remains small, only 1 in 83,000.[1]

Given this medical evidence, one next needs to articulate the values that are in conflict. The first is the patient's right to know the risks of any given procedure. Many argue that HIV infection is a real even though improbable risk. Certainly the greater the magnitude or severity of the risk, the greater the obligation to disclose it. Although patients are exposed constantly to various sources of nosocomial infection without being informed, the case of HIV infection differs in that the risk for the patient theoretically can be eliminated by choosing a noninfected health care professional. When disclosing risks, the health care professional usually is held to the standard of revealing what a reasonable person would want to know. Does the fact that most people, including health care professionals, want to know the HIV status of their physician suggest a standard of reasonableness? Should not the patient be fully informed and then determine what is an acceptable risk? Second, health care professionals value their obligation not to subject their patients to avoidable harms. Ethicists recognize the duty to warn people and reveal sensitive information when it can prevent serious harm, when there is no other way of preventing the harm, and when the disclosure of information will not result in even greater harm.

In contrast, several considerations mitigate against the testing of health care professionals and disclosure of HIV status. First, because of societal discrimination, disclosure of HIV status has led and will continue to lead to the destruction of professionals' careers as well as lives. Maintaining appropriate confidentiality often emerges as a difficult if not impossible task. Second, if disclosure will lead to a destruction of a professional's practice, then professionals may avoid subjecting themselves to the risk of infection. Specifically they will become reluctant to treat HIV infected patients. Moreover, they will call more vociferously for mandatory testing of patients to minimize exposure to HIV. Third, this will lead subsequently to an even more adversarial relationship between health care professionals and patients because each will see the other as a threat to life, health, and career. At a time when the fiduciary nature of this relationship is strained, mandatory testing of health care workers would serve only to exacerbate the problem. Fourth, in an age of exorbitant and uncontrolled health care costs, testing would be prohibitively expensive. One would have to test workers continually to ensure safety, yet at what intervals—every day, every week, every month, every year? Furthermore, because a worker could seroconvert at any time and the AIDS test has the possibility of false negatives, a patient could never be fully confident that the health care worker was indeed HIV negative.

DISCUSSION

In Congressional hearings, many "reasonable" people supported Kimberly Bergalis (a patient of Dr. Acer who developed AIDS) in her call for testing of health care workers. Nevertheless, current scientific data does not seem to justify the disclosure of HIV status. Patients do not inquire about other risks even though the risk to life and health could be significant. For example, patients do not investigate how much sleep doctors had the night before surgery, their alcohol consumption patterns, or their Hepatitis B status. Hence, the desire to ascertain HIV status appears to be more a manifestation of irrational fears associated with AIDS hysteria than a "reasonable" standard for informed consent. Moreover, because the risk for transmission is so small, the health care professional does not have a duty to warn, especially because measures are available to prevent infection through universal precautions. It may be argued that surgeons still cut themselves during surgery despite precautions. However, because the risk of transmission is so negligible, testing and disclosure seems to be an exaggerated response. Additionally, the detriments of testing, which include its impracticality, its prohibitive costs, and its debilitative effect on the patient/health care professional relationship, outweigh the minimal potential for preventing transmission. Thus, sometimes, other goods take precedence over the individual's right to know.

Nevertheless, health care professionals may and perhaps should choose to be tested voluntarily if they engage in actions that make them susceptible to infection. The reason for this is not primarily to prevent the spread of HIV infection to the patient. Rather, health care professionals may want to know their status for early prophylaxis and to be alert for signs and symptoms that could compromise patient care, especially as the disease progresses towards full-blown AIDS. In such cases the health care worker will be susceptible to opportunistic diseases like TB, which could be more easily passed on to unwitting patients. Furthermore, AIDS dementia may affect memory and judgment, which may require close monitoring, again for patient safety. Thus, it would seem appropriate to set up confidential review committees in institutions that could counsel workers on a case-by-case basis when to refrain from certain practices, not because of fear of transmitting HIV infection but because of a diminution in professional ability. Health care workers who are in fact HIV positive may choose in conscience to refrain from certain exposure prone procedures and may divulge their HIV status to patients voluntarily. However, this should not be mandated unless new empirical data on the possibility of transmission emerges.

CONCLUSION

The clamor for testing of health care workers (especially physicians, and, more specifically, surgeons) will continue in the general public. Administrators may support such measures because of concern about legal liability. However, legislative and internal policy measures to follow through on these proposals should be resisted at this time. Current scientific evidence does not substantiate the need for broad-scale testing, disclosure of HIV status, or immediate restriction of the practice of professionals. The use and enforcement of universal precautions should provide sufficient protection at a much lower cost. Moreover, proposals for testing are likely to cause more harm than good, adversely affecting the patient/health care professional relationship. This may result eventually in greater harm for patients because of professional's reluctance to treat anyone that might be a threat to his or her career.

NOTE

1. A. Lowenfels and G. Wormser, "Risk of Transmission of HIV from Surgeon to Patient," *New England Journal of Medicine,* 325 (1991): 888–89.

71: Separating the Lakeberg Twins: Ethical Issues

Amy and Angela Lakeberg were born on June 29, 1993, at Loyola University Medical Center in Maywood, Illinois, a suburb of Chicago. Before their birth, their parents learned that the twins were joined at the chest. Upon delivery, they learned that the twins shared a heart and liver. In the opinion of the neonatal physicians at Loyola, both would soon die if they were not separated. Moreover, even if they were separated, the chance of keeping the surviving twin alive was reckoned at "less than 1 percent." The parents, after being informed by the Loyola physicians of the situation, requested to have the twins separated, in hopes one would survive. Accordingly, a surgical team from Children's Hospital in Philadelphia, which had operated on several other sets of conjoined twins in recent years, agreed to accept the case. Surgery was performed in Philadelphia in August 1993. As a result of the effort to position a functioning heart in the body of one of the twins, Amy died and Angela still survives, albeit on a respirator. After delivery, and before and after the surgery to separate the twins, a discussion was carried on in the media concerning the ethical issues arising from the Lakeberg case. In this essay, we shall consider these issues.

EFFECTIVE SURGERY?

It seems the first ethical issue in the Lakeberg case is whether or not to perform surgery. Moreover, it seems we have to evaluate the surgery both as therapy and as a research project. Insofar as therapy is concerned, surgery should be performed if it is judged effective and does not impose a grave burden. Surgery is effective if it will enable the patient, in this case the twins, to pursue the purpose of life. That is, will the surgery enable the twins to think, love, relate to others and to pursue the goods of life which are associated with human fulfillment? Clearly, surgery alone will not help a person strive for the purpose of life, but surgery can establish a physiological basis for this endeavor. In answering this question concerning the effectiveness of the surgery, we are faced immediately with the realization that one of the twins will die as a result of the surgery. Thus, the surgery would not be effective insofar as the non-surviving twin was concerned. Because it was foreseen that Amy would die, some people condemned the surgery because they said it would involve killing Amy in order to save Angela. It seems on the other hand, that this is a classic case of the principle of double effect. The object of the moral action is to save Angela through surgery, and in the course of performing this action, because of the position of the shared organs, an unwanted effect occurs necessarily, namely the death of Amy. From the point of view of Amy's death then, it does not seem that the surgery involves a direct killing.

Is the surgery effective from the point of view of Angela? This is difficult to answer because her prognosis is so uncertain. The neonatologists at Loyola and the surgeons in Philadelphia did not offer much more hope of success than 1 percent. That means a 99 percent chance of failure. And we have no idea of what the possibility of "success" implied. Would it be considered a successful surgery if Angela merely survived after the surgery for a few weeks or months? Would the surgery be successful if Angela were to be respirator dependent for years to come and need to remain in an institution? How would neurological deficit be reckoned insofar as success in concerned? Though it is difficult to determine the meaning of "success" insofar as the surgery is concerned, given the uncertainty of Angela's survival for any length of time, and given the debilitated condition which would probably ensue after surgery, it seems a bit optimistic to say that the surgery had a 1% chance of success.

EXCESSIVE BURDEN?

Even if some would judge the surgery to be potentially effective for Angela, it must also be evaluated insofar as the burden it imposes is concerned. The burden of any medical therapy must be considered from the point of view of the patient, and also from the point of view of the family and society. When we consider the burden from the point of view of Angela, we consider not only the burden of the surgery, but also the burden that will be imposed upon her in the future as a result of the surgery. In regard to the surgery itself, it doesn't seem to have imposed an excessive burden upon Angela. But did the surgery impose an excessive burden insofar as Angela's future life is concerned? This is difficult to decide because of the vagueness of the prognosis and the uncertainty of her function and survival. Even if the surgery allows Angela to survive, will it be a beneficial survival, or a burdensome survival? At the time of the surgery, no one could say. But how many ventures would a prudent person pursue, if the hope for success were less than 1%? Can the burden be deemed excessive insofar as the parents are concerned? Reitha and Ken seemed willing to assume the burden associated with caring for Angela. Hence it would be difficult to assert excessive burden insofar as the parents are concerned. Insofar as society is concerned, the main objection to the surgery concerned the money that would be spent upon the care of the twins in the tertiary care facilities in Maywood and Philadelphia. The statement was often made, "Couldn't that money be put to better use; for example, by devoting it to prenatal care?" The fact is, that if the money were not devoted to the care of the twins, it would not be devoted to prenatal care. Our society has a very convoluted method of funding health care for catastrophic cases like the Lakebergs. Funding of health care results from an amalgam of public, private, and charitable sources, which are unpredictable, but which often provide the necessary funds. While this does not seem to be the optimal method of funding health care, nonetheless, it is the method that exists in our society at present. Thus, it doesn't seem that physicians and hospital administrators who cared for the Lakeberg twins can be faulted for a misuse of resources once they decided to perform the surgery. The surgeon in Philadelphia seems to be justified in saying: "If someone is going to ration health care because of money, it is not going to be us." In the future, society may wish to address the economic implications of catastrophic treatment in a more reasonable manner, but at present, surgeons do not have the responsibility of allocating funds for catastrophic cases.

RESEARCH

If the surgery were deemed ineffective or excessively burdensome as a medical procedure, could it be justified as a research project? Research, in the strict sense of the term, does not aim at healing or curing, but rather at acquiring new knowledge for the good of humanity. Of course, research is often combined with therapy, and then the overall project does have a healing or curing purpose. But in the strict sense, research seeks to gain knowledge that will benefit people in the future. One can accept serious risk of harm for oneself and thus volunteer for research projects in the strict sense of the term. But the ethical validity of proxy consent does not allow one person to put another person at risk of serious harm unless there is hope of therapeutic benefit. When the ethical issues of the Lakeberg case were discussed, some expressed the thought that the surgery was justified because it might provide knowledge for the future. But the risk to the twins was too great, especially to Amy, to justify the surgery under the title of research. The history of research upon humans, from Auschwitz to Tuskeegee, is replete with examples of both subjects and researchers being dehumanized as a result of research without informed consent.

DECISION MAKERS

Finally, who has the ethical right and responsibility to make decisions concerning the medical care of the Lakeberg twins? The first response to this question might be "the parents" because the children are not able to offer consent for themselves. However, this response is a bit shortsighted because when making any type of reasonable decision parents will require medical information from the physicians involved in the case. Thus, informed consent, especially in the case of infants, is a collaborative decision. The physicians must make a decision whether or not the surgery would seem to be effective and offer this information to the parents. Insofar as ethical medicine is concerned, the physicians have the right and often the obligation to declare that a particular therapy is futile, and that they do not offer that particular therapy as an option. Unfortunately, in the United States at this time, physicians seldom make a declaration that a particular therapy is futile if the parents or proxies of incapacitated patients vehemently request such therapy. The mentality of the physicians in the Lakeberg case was evidenced by a surgeon in Philadelphia who stated that the main reason for performing the surgery was the Lakeberg's wishes. "We take the position that the parents have the right to choose for their children." This is true, in most cases, but not if the surgery is ineffective in the minds of the surgeons. A more collaborative decision might have yielded a different decision in the Lakeberg case.

CONCLUSION

The most disconcerting aspect of the Lakeberg case is the realization that ethical decisions often must be made with incomplete and insufficient information. When this happens, there is no moral mandate to pursue the course of action which might prolong life, especially if there is only insignificant hope of success. As Daniel Callahan remarks: "The yoking of sanctity of life and the technological imperative has led to the common conclusion that, when in doubt, we should treat." But the ethical reality is that actions need not be performed if the hope of success is very remote. Hence, there is no ethical mandate to do whatever is possible, rather there is a mandate to do what is reasonable. With this in mind, not because millions of dollars were expended, it seems the decisions made to separate the Lakeberg twins may be called into question.

Index

ABOUT THE AUTHORS

Jean deBlois, CSJ, born in San Francisco, California, earned the PhD in moral theology at the Catholic University of America. She is a former staff member of the Center for Health Care Ethics. At present, she serves as senior associate, clinical ethics, The Catholic Health Association, St. Louis, Missouri.

Patrick Norris, OP, a native of Albuquerque, New Mexico is a member of the Dominican Order, Central Province. He is associate director of the Center for Health Care Ethics, an instructor in medical ethics, department of internal medicine, Saint Louis University Health Sciences Center, and a candidate for the PhD in theology, St. Louis University.

Kevin O'Rourke, OP, a native of Park Ridge, Illinois is a member of the Dominican Order, Central Province. He is professor of medical ethics, School of Medicine, St. Louis University Health Sciences Center, and director of the Center for Health Care Ethics. He earned a doctorate in canon law at St. Thomas University in Rome and has been awarded the Master of Theology Degree by the Dominican Order.